Human Fertility
Reproductive Biology

Akmal El-Mazny

Copyright © 2019 Akmal El-Mazny

All rights reserved.

Amazon KDP, USA

ISBN: 9781792651175

Contents

	Page
Introduction	1
FEMALE REPRODUCTIVE BIOLOGY	2
Ovaries	3
Hormonal Control	6
Ovarian Cycle	14
Oocyte Development	20
– Ovarian Factors of Infertility	25
Fallopian Tubes	28
Fertilization	31
– Tubal Factors of Infertility	33
Uterus	37
Endometrial Cycle	41
Implantation	44
Embryo Development	45
– Uterine Factors of Infertility	48
Cervix	52
Capacitation	54
– Cervical Factors of Infertility	55
MALE REPRODUCTIVE BIOLOGY	56
Hormonal Control	57
– Pretesticular Factors of Infertility	59
Testes	60
Spermatogenesis	65
– Testicular Factors of Infertility	70
Duct System	75
Accessory Glands	83
Penis	88
Erection and Ejaculation	92
– Posttesticular Factors of Infertility	94
References	96

INTRODUCTION

The functions of the reproductive system are to produce and deliver gametes (spermatozoa or oocytes) for sexual reproduction, and produce hormones that regulate reproductive function.

Abnormalities in the physiologic function affect the development and delivery of gametes, and potential fertility.

Female infertility can be divided into several categories: ovarian, tubal, uterine, cervical, and other.

Male infertility may be due to abnormalities of hormonal control, testicular function, or sperm transport.

This book provides a comprehensive review of human reproductive biology; emphasizing hormonal control, gamete production, fertilization, implantation, and embryonic development.

By developing a clear understanding of what is normal, you will better understand the abnormalities affecting fertility and the mechanisms behind treatment.

FEMALE REPRODUCTIVE BIOLOGY

The female reproductive system is a complicated but fascinating subject.

It has the capability to function intimately with nearly every other body system for the purpose of reproduction.

The female reproductive system consists of the hypothalamic-pituitary unit, the ovaries, the reproductive tract, and the external genitalia.

The functions of the female reproductive system are to produce and deliver oocytes, for sexual reproduction, and produce hormones that regulate reproductive function and secondary sex characteristics.

The female reproductive organs can be subdivided into the internal and external genitalia.

The internal genitalia are those organs that are within the true pelvis: the ovaries, fallopian tubes, uterus, cervix, and vagina.

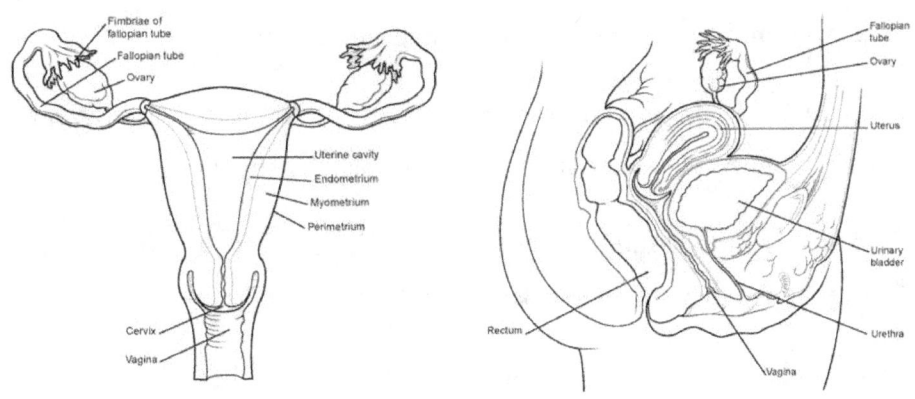

Female Reproductive System

OVARIES

The ovaries are paired organs located on either side of the uterus within the mesovarium portion of the broad ligament below the uterine tubes.

At birth, a female has approximately 1-2 million eggs, but only 300 of these eggs ever mature and are released for the purpose of fertilization.

The ovaries are small and oval-shaped, exhibit a grayish color, and have an uneven surface.

The actual size of an ovary depends on a woman's age and hormonal status; the ovaries are approximately 3-5 cm in length during childbearing years and become much smaller and atrophic once menopause occurs.

A cross-section of the ovary reveals many cystic structures that vary in size representing ovarian follicles at different stages of development and degeneration.

Several ligaments support the ovary:

– The ovarian ligament connects the uterus and ovary.

– The posterior portion of the broad ligament forms the mesovarium, which supports the ovary and houses the vascular supply.

– The suspensory (infundibular) ligament of the ovary, a peritoneal fold overlying the ovarian vessels, attaches the ovary to the pelvic side wall.

Blood supply to the ovary is via the ovarian artery; both right and left ovarian arteries originate directly from the descending aorta at the level of the L2 vertebra, and enter the ovary at the hilum.

The left ovarian vein drains into the left renal vein, and the right ovarian vein empties directly into the inferior vena cava.

Lymphatic drainage of the ovary is primarily to the lateral aortic nodes; however, the iliac nodes may also be involved.

Nerve supply to the ovaries, through the ovarian, hypogastric, and aortic plexuses, run with the vasculature within the suspensory ligament of the ovary entering the ovary at the hilum.

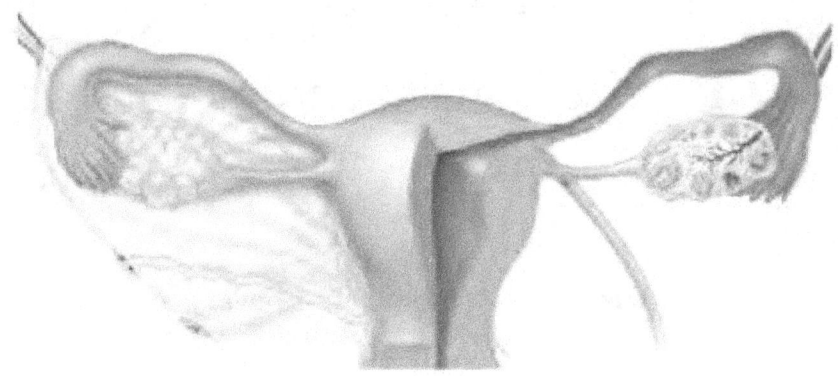

Gross Anatomy of the Ovaries

Microscopic Anatomy

The ovaries are covered externally by a layer of simple cuboidal epithelium called germinal (ovarian) epithelium.

Beneath this layer is a dense connective tissue capsule, the tunica albuginea.

The main body of the ovary is divided into an outer cortex and an inner medulla.

- The cortex is dense and granular and contains numerous ovarian follicles in various stages of development.

- The medulla is loose connective tissue with abundant blood vessels, lymphatic vessels, and nerve fibers.

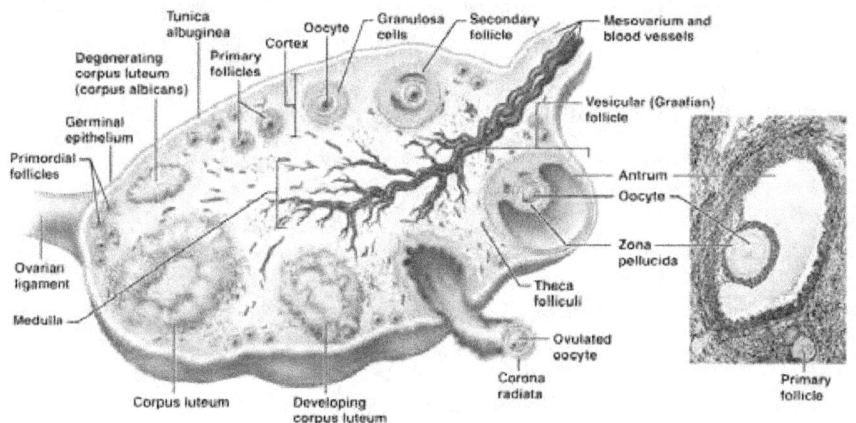

Microscopic Anatomy of the Ovary

Functions

- The ovary cyclically produces gametes; the number of oocytes (germ cells) available is determined during fetal development and continues to decline by either ovulation or atresia until menopause occurs.

- It also cyclically secretes hormones (androgens, estrogens, progestins) that prepare the reproductive tract for oocyte transport, fertilization, implantation and pregnancy, and it controls the hypothalamic-pituitary unit through negative and positive feedback mechanisms.

HORMONAL CONTROL

There are four major functional compartments involved in reproduction, each has a specific function: the hypothalamus, the pituitary gland and the ovaries, which compose the hypothalamic-pituitary-ovarian (HPO) axis; and the hormonally-responsive functional endometrium lining the uterus.

In the presence of low levels of estrogen, the arcuate nucleus of the hypothalamus releases gonadotropin-releasing hormone.

This hormone signals the anterior pituitary to produce the gonadotropins LH and FSH.

These gonadotropins in turn induce the development and maturation of ovarian follicles that contain the actual oocytes.

During the growth process, the follicles produce increased amounts of estradiol.

This increase in estrogen production develops the endometrium and thins the increasing amounts of cervical mucus.

When the estradiol level reaches an appropriate level, generally when the follicle is mature, the pituitary releases a large amount of LH.

LH surge causes the final maturation of the oocyte and stimulates the event of ovulation.

After the oocyte is released, that is, ovulation occurs, the sac containing the oocyte undergoes metamorphosis with growth of new blood vessels and becomes a functioning gland called the corpus luteum.

The corpus luteum produces progesterone in large amounts and estrogen in smaller amounts.

Progesterone stabilizes the endometrium and thickens the cervical mucus.

The lifespan of corpus luteum is about 14 days, unless pregnancy occurs.

If the woman does not conceive in a particular cycle, after 14 days, the corpus luteum stops producing progesterone, the endometrium is no longer stable, and menses begin.

The normal menstrual cycle length is 25 to 35 days; this cyclicity is determined by changing sensitivities of the hypothalamic-pituitary unit to estrogens and progestins.

The HPO axis also involves a negative feedback loop in which gonadal secretions produced in response to pituitary gonadotropins inhibit further secretion of gonadotropins.

The HPO axis in the female also involves a positive feedback loop in which ovarian estrogen produced in response to pituitary FSH enhances pituitary secretion of LH and FSH.

Functional Compartment	Location	Hormone or Function
- Hypothalamus	- Arcuate nucleus	- GnRH
- Anterior pituitary	- Gonadotropin	- FSH
		- LH
- Ovary	- Follicle	- Estradiol
	- Corpus luteum	- Progesterone
		- Inhibin
		- Activin
		- Anti-Mullerian hormone
- Uterus	- Endometrium	- Proliferative
		- Secretory
		- Menses

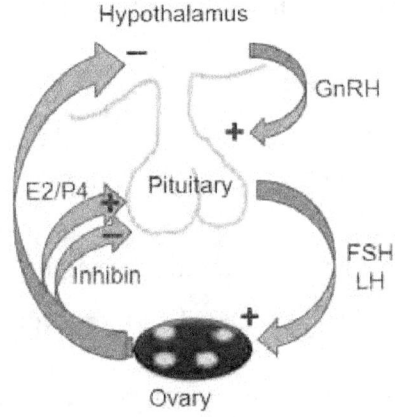

Hypothalamic-Pituitary-Ovarian (HPO) Axis

Hypothalamus - GnRH

GnRH is synthesized and secreted by neurons in the arcuate nucleus of the hypothalamus and diffuses into the hypothalamic-hypophyseal portal vessels, which transport it to the anterior pituitary gland.

Through pulsatile release, GnRH stimulates the gonadotropes to produce FSH and LH.

The activity of this decapeptide can be modified by changing one or more amino acids; this creates GnRH agonists or antagonists that are often used as adjuncts to infertility and other medical disorders.

Anterior Pituitary - FSH

FSH is a heterodimeric glycoprotein synthesized in gonadotropes in the anterior pituitary.

It has a relatively long half-life in the plasma, normally 3-4 hours; peripheral plasma levels of FSH do not reflect pulsatile GnRH secretion.

FSH stimulates granulosa cells of the ovarian follicle and the luteinized cells of the corpus luteum.

It is considered the critical regulator of follicular development because it is capable of stimulating follicular development by itself.

FSH is suppressed by rising estradiol from the growing follicle; cyclic levels are at their maximum on Day 3 and midcycle surge.

The number of primary follicles which begin to enlarge and respond to FSH is related to the age and total number of oocytes present in the ovary.

Since there is no maturing follicle to suppress FSH, during menopause, FSH is elevated.

Anterior Pituitary - LH

LH is a heterodimeric glycoprotein synthesized in the same gonadotropes in the anterior pituitary as FSH.

LH has a shorter plasma half life (about 20 minutes) than FSH, so peripheral plasma levels do reflect the pronounced pulsatile pattern of GnRH secretion.

LH is secreted in a pulsatile manner:

– In the follicular phase, the pulse interval is normally 90 min.

– In the luteal phase it is about 2 to 3 hours.

LH stimulates mature granulosa cells of the preovulatory follicle and their successor cells, the luteinized cells of the corpus luteum.

LH is capable of maintaining the lifespan of the corpus luteum beyond the normal luteal phase of the menstrual cycle; however, LH is rapidly degraded when administered by injection.

HCG mimics LH, and can therefore stimulate ovulation and support the luteal phase; hCG has a much longer half life and is slower to degrade when administered by injection.

LH has the following stimulatory effects on ovarian cells:

– Increases availability of free cholesterol.

– Stimulates production of androgens in ovarian theca and interstitial cells by increasing enzymes for androgen biosynthesis.

– Increases production of progesterone and estradiol in the corpus luteum.

– Increases plasminogen activator synthesis and secretion in granulosa cells of the preovulatory follicle.

– Stimulates resumption of meiosis in the oocyte at midcycle.

Ovary - Sex Steroids

Although the ovary secretes many substances steroid hormones including androgens, estrogens and progestins, appear to be among the most important.

Androgens are synthesized in the theca and interstitial cells and are important as substrates for estrogen biosynthesis.

The adrenal glands are the principal source of circulating androgens (dehydroepiandrosterone, androstenedione, and testosterone) in women.

The increase in synthesis of adrenal androgens at puberty (called adrenarche) stimulates the development of axillary, pubic and facial hair.

High levels of androgens suppress progesterone synthesis in granulosa cells.

Although the ovaries and adrenals produce similar quantities of androstenedione and testosterone, most of the ovarian androgens are converted to estrogens in the ovaries and in peripheral tissues.

Most of the testosterone in the plasma of the adult female is formed by peripheral conversion of androstenedione by peripheral 17β-hydroxysteroid dehydrogenase.

Estradiol is considered the most important product of the granulosa cells of the developing follicle; estrone is a less active estrogen than estradiol.

Estradiol concentrations in plasma reach a peak during the late follicular phase, decline after ovulation and then rise again during the luteal phase.

Progesterone is considered the most important product of the corpus luteum.

Ovary - Inhibins and Activins

Inhibin is a heterodimeric glycoprotein consisting of an alpha and a beta subunit and is synthesized by granulosa and luteal cells of the ovary.

FSH stimulates granulosa cells to synthesize and secrete inhibin, so that as follicles enlarge, they produce increasing amounts of the hormone.

Inhibin preferentially inhibits synthesis and secretion of FSH but not LH by pituitary gonadotropes (negative feedback).

Inhibin production is low at the beginning of the menstrual cycle, then increases late in the follicular phase and reaches a peak prior to the preovulatory surge of FSH and LH.

After ovulation, inhibin levels decrease slightly, followed by a final rise in the midluteal phase to a level twice that at midcycle.

As the corpus luteum regresses, inhibin levels decline and FSH levels rise with the beginning of the next menstrual cycle.

The ovarian granulosa cells also secrete activin, a dimeric protein consisting of two of the β subunits of inhibin.

Activin amplifies the effect of FSH on granulosa cells in the ovary and also increases the synthesis of the FSH β subunit in the anterior pituitary.

Neuroendocrine Control

– Inhibin, acts on the pituitary to suppress the synthesis and release of FSH, but does not impact LH.

– In the follicular phase, estrogen exerts negative feedback by decreasing the pulse amplitude thereby decreasing FSH and LH pulse amplitude.

– In the luteal phase, progesterone and testosterone decrease GnRH pulse frequency resulting in decreased FSH and LH pulse frequency.

– Testosterone inhibits gonadotropin gene expression in the anterior pituitary; women with elevated serum testosterone levels often do not have normal menstrual cycles.

– GnRH is also inhibited by high concentrations of prolactin; breastfeeding may act as a contraceptive.

- The thyroid can also impact the HPO axis; thyrotropin-releasing hormone (TRH) at high concentrations stimulates the pituitary gland to produce prolactin; patients with hypothyroidism or secondary hyperthyroidism also have decreased gonadotropin secretion.

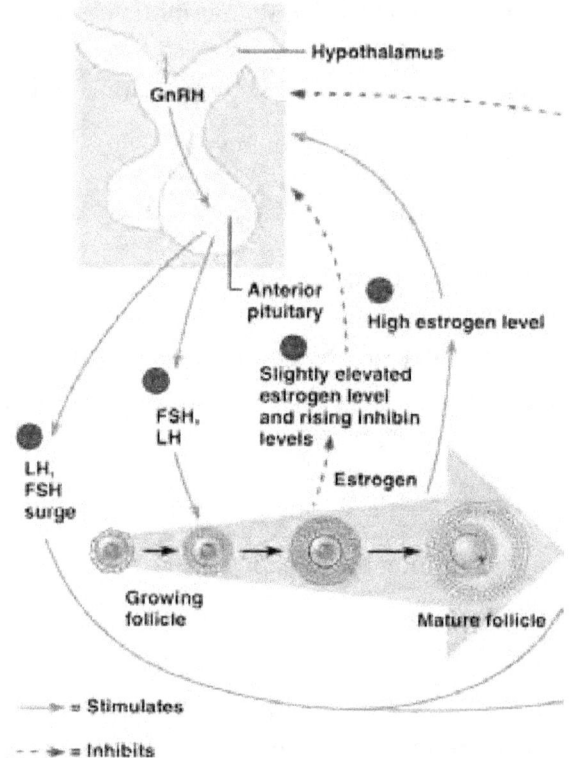

Neuroendocrine Control

OVARIAN CYCLE

The follicle is the basic functional unit of the ovary.

Each follicle consists of an oocyte surrounded by one or more layers of specialized cells (granulosa, theca) which secrete autocrine, paracrine, and endocrine factors.

The follicle grows under the influence of gonadotropins (FSH, LH) and intraovarian regulators (estradiol, IGF-I, activin).

Development from a primordial follicle to a preovulatory follicle takes three to four menstrual cycles.

Follicular Phase

Primordial Follicle

— Primordial follicles are formed during fetal life and are not believed to require gonadotropins for formation; however, females lacking functional FSH receptors have poorly developed ovaries.

— A primordial follicle consists of an oocyte and a single layer of epithelial cells.

— The oocyte is arrested in the first meiotic prophase.

— During the first cycle of development the oocyte grows to about 100 microns in diameter and the epithelial cells enlarge and become cuboidal granulosa cells; at this point, the oocyte is referred to as the "primary follicle".

— FSH receptors are first detectable on the plasma membrane of granulosa cells.

— The granulosa cells respond to FSH by proliferating faster.

Preantral Follicle

— During the first to second cycles of development, the primary follicle progresses to the preantral stage.

— Oocyte meiosis remains arrested.

— The oocyte completes the first step of meiotic maturation, which includes germinal vesicle breakdown and metaphase I after the mid-cycle LH surge.

— Preantral follicles respond to the midcycle surge of FSH during the second to third cycles of development by growing rapidly; this event is called recruitment.

— All recruited follicles produce sex steroid hormones in amounts proportional to their size and degree of maturation.

— A single follicle, the most mature follicle, becomes dominant.

— The remaining follicles degenerate through a process called atresia.

— The emergence of the single dominant follicle appears to result from the inhibin-induced decline in plasma FSH concentrations.

— Once a dominant follicle is selected, rising serum hormone levels of inhibin and estradiol suppress FSH.

− Local production of estradiol by the dominant follicle amplifies the response to FSH.

− Estradiol synthesis continues to increase exponentially in response to FSH.

Antral Follicle

− Fluid accumulates among the granulosa cells forming the antrum.

− After the antrum is formed, the follicle is termed a "secondary follicle".

Preovulatory Follicle

− During the last cycle of development (third or fourth cycle), the dominant follicle attains its maximal size and the theca layer vascularizes; this represents the "Graafian follicle".

− The oocyte (meiosis still arrested) has the capacity to proceed to metaphase II and complete meiotic maturation after fertilization.

− Granulosa cells of immature follicles have few LH receptors so they don't respond to LH at physiological LH concentrations.

− The theca cells do have LH receptors and they respond to LH.

− One of the actions of FSH on granulosa cells during the follicular phase is to induce LH receptors so that granulosa cells of the preovulatory Graafian follicle become responsive to LH as well as to FSH.

− After the LH/FSH surge prior to ovulation, the granulosa cells initially decrease their LH and FSH receptors and then increase them as the granulosa cells luteinize to become the corpus luteum.

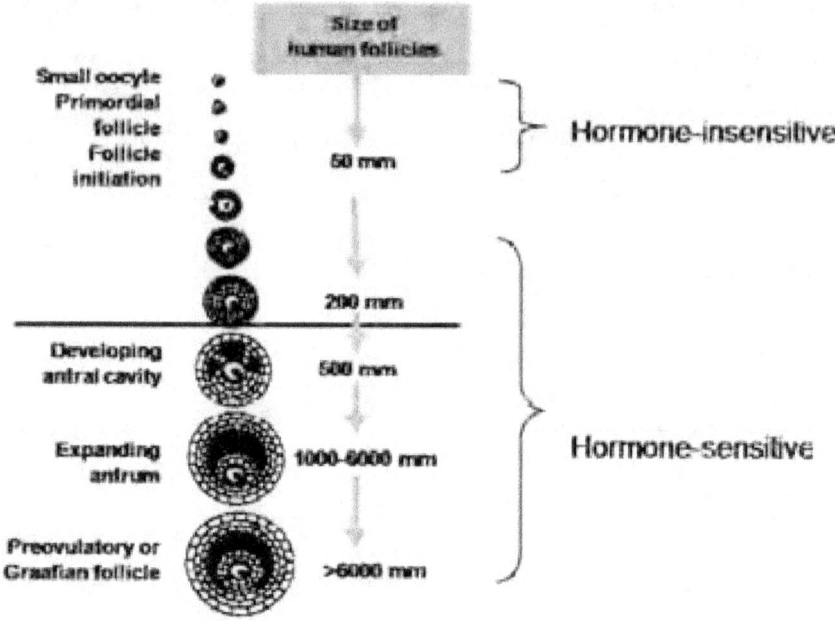

Follicle Development

Ovulation Phase

– LH triggers several processes that culminate in ovulation.

– LH causes a resumption of oocyte meiosis, and metaphase I is completed.

– The first polar body is extruded, and meiosis then halts in metaphase II.

– An increase in follicular pressure, combined with LH-activated breakdown of the follicular wall results in follicular rupture.

– The cumulus-oocyte complex is ovulated 34-36 hours after the onset of the LH surge, and the remaining granulosa and theca cells luteinize.

Luteal Phase

– After ovulation the follicular cells luteinize and form the corpus luteum (literally, yellow body).

– They acquire the capacity to secrete progesterone, and lipid droplets accumulate in the cells.

– If the oocyte is fertilized and implants in the endometrium, the corpus luteum remains active and secretes progesterone in large amounts and estradiol in smaller amounts.

– Progesterone from the corpus luteum prepares the endometrium for implantation and maintains the fetal-placental unit during the first half of the first trimester of pregnancy.

– The corpus luteum requires low levels of LH for continued function.

– LH stimulates the production of progesterone and estradiol, and FSH stimulates the production of estradiol only.

– If fertilization and implantation do not occur, the corpus luteum degenerates (called luteolysis), and progesterone declines within 10 days after ovulation.

– Unlike the variable length of the follicular phase of the menstrual cycle, the luteal phase has a lifespan of about 14 days; this lifespan is due to the fairly consistent lifespan of the corpus luteum.

– However, if pregnancy occurs, the corpus luteum is rescued by hCG that is produced by the implanted trophoblasts.

- LH and hCG are similar in structure; hCG may be thought of as long acting LH.

- In clinical situations hCG injections are used to act like LH, particularly to induce ovulation or stimulate luteal progesterone production.

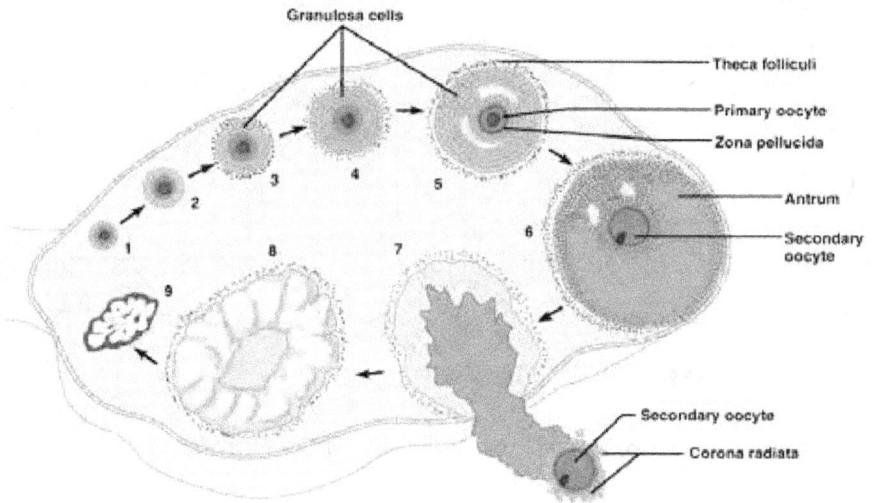

Ovarian Cycle

OOCYTE DEVELOPMENT

The ovaries and germ cells (which develop into oocytes) form during the first few weeks of embryonic life.

These germ cells rapidly divide by a process called mitosis, in which each new daughter cell contains the same number of chromosomes as the parent cell.

During the first trimester of embryonic growth, these preoocyte cells are called oogonium (plural: oogonia).

During the second trimester of life, the 46 chromosomes start to replicate through the process of meiosis but remain within the cell.

At this stage of meiosis, the cell is called a primary oocyte (primitive ovum not yet fully developed).

At this point, further chromosome separation and oocyte development are arrested until after puberty.

These primary oocytes are surrounded by a layer of epithelium that gives rise to the primordial follicles.

About 1700 germ cells are present before migration to the genital ridge begins.

However, these multiply during the process of migration, reaching a peak of 7 million oocytes at midgestation.

The primordial germ cells increase in size early in their development and become oogonia.

At midgestation, they begin the first meiotic division, becoming primary oocytes.

This prophase lasts until just before ovulation, which may occur 12 to 40 or more years later.

In this state, they are no longer capable of multiplication and, in fact, steadily decline in number.

About 400 ova are released through the process of ovulation during a woman's lifetime.

The remaining ova undergo atresia (a normal process affecting the primordial ovarian follicles in which death of the ovum results in degeneration) so that, by the time of the menopause, few are present.

The oocyte remains in this stage until it is either eliminated by atresia or succeeds in reaching the maturation stage and resumption of meiosis (reduction division) at the time of ovulation.

Meiosis has two purposes: reduction to the haploid number of chromosomes to one half of the normal, or 23, and recombination of genetic information.

The first meiotic division, which begins during fetal life, is completed prior to ovulation and produces a secondary oocyte containing 23 chromosomes and the first polar body containing 23 chromosomes, each with 2 daughter chromatids.

A polar body is composed of cell division products that result from meiosis.

The second meiotic division, which is initiated after ovulation, is completed at sperm penetration and produces a mature oocyte containing 23 chromosomes and a polar body containing 23 chromosomes, each with a single chromatid.

When the oocyte and sperm combine at fertilization, the full complement of 46 chromosomes is restored and a new life is created.

The second polar body will degenerate like the first.

As a result of the combined meiotic processes, a single mature oocyte is produced and 2 or 3 polar bodies degenerate.

This is in contrast to the meiotic process in males where a single precursor cell gives rise to 4 mature sperm.

Oocyte Maturation and Ovulation

– Resumption of meiosis begins within the ovarian follicle in response to the LH surge.

– The granulosa cells, that is, the cumulus oophorus, expands.

– The first polar body is extruded and the oocyte progresses into metaphase of the second meiotic division.

– Meiosis stops in metaphase II until fertilization.

Fertilization

Contractions of the oviductal muscles direct the oocyte into the ampulla of the fallopian tube where it remains for about 3 days while the ampullary-isthmic sphincter remains contracted.

The oocytes remain fertile for only 15-18 hours after ovulation while sperm are motile for 24 hours to several days after ejaculation.

When a sperm encounters the zona pellucida, it undergoes an acrosome reaction; this breaks down the acrosomal membrane.

The sperm head membrane binds to the sperm receptor, which is followed by fusion with the oolemma.

Microvilli on the oocyte surface surround the sperm head and the oocyte undergoes the cortical reaction (release of cortical granules).

The zona pellucida hardens and no other sperm can penetrate the oolemma.

The oocyte nucleus completes maturation to yield the female pronucleus and the second polar body; the sperm nucleus forms the male pronucleus.

The corona radiata is the layer of granulosa cells surrounding the oocyte; the zona pellucida is an extracellular layer of proteins surrounding the oocyte.

Egg Activation

Egg activation occurs after fertilization, and involves the completion of the second meiotic division and initiation of embryonic development.

Mitosis begins and there are changes in maternal messenger ribonucleic acids and protein synthesis.

Exocytosis of cortical granules blocks polyspermy and cytoskeletal rearrangement occurs.

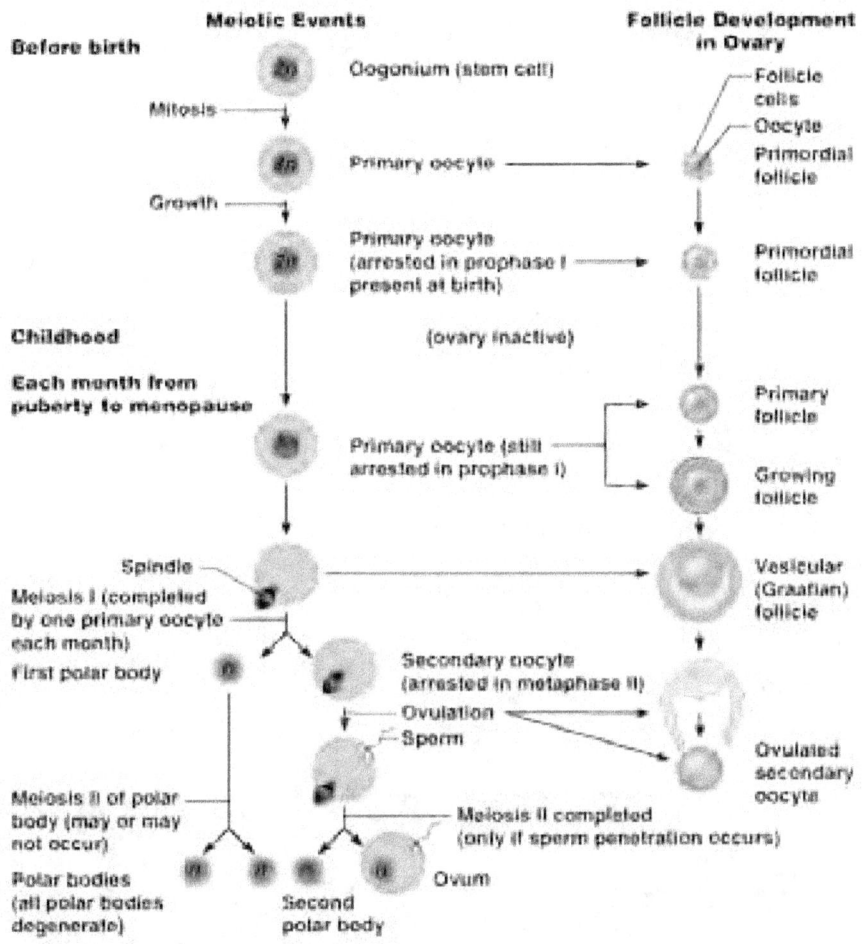

Oocyte Development

OVARIAN FACTORS OF INFERTILITY

Causes

Alteration in the frequency and duration of the menstrual cycle.

Failure to ovulate is the most common infertility problem

− Polycystic ovarian syndrome (PCOS).

− Hypergonadotropic hypogonadism.

− Hypogonadotropic hypogonadism.

− Prolactin disorders.

− Chromosomal abnormalities.

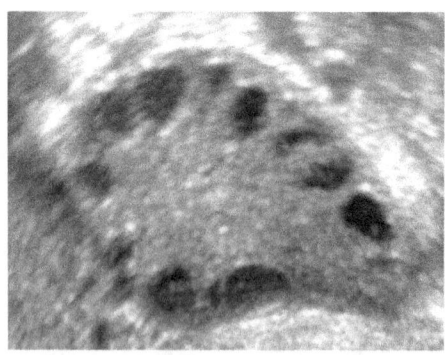   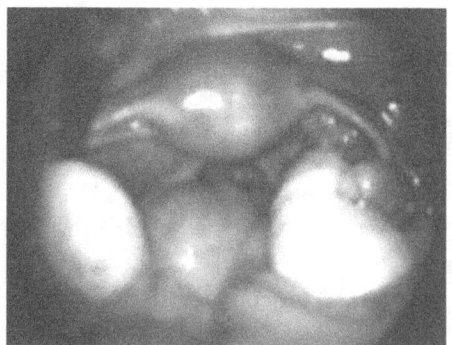

Ultrasonography   **Laparoscopy**

Polycystic Ovarian Syndrome (PCOS)

Investigations

Progesterone levels and ultrasonography to assess ovulation; LH/FSH ratio to assess PCOS; FSH and estradiol levels (or antral follicle count, ovarian volume, and AMH) to assess ovarian reserve; clomiphene citrate challenge test for dynamic ovarian reserve testing.

Treatment

Treatment of ovarian factors may be medical (eg, pharmacotherapy) or surgical (eg, ovarian drilling).

Induction of Ovulation

Ovulation induction is the appropriate treatment for infertile patients who have dysfunction of the hypothalamic-pituitary-ovarian axis.

−Clomiphene Citrate (CC)

−Tamoxifen

−Aromatase Inhibitors

−Dopamine Agonists

−Human Menopausal Gonadotropins (hMG)

−Human Chorionic Gonadotropins (hCG)

−Gonadotropin Releasing Hormone (GnRH)

−Gonadotropin Releasing Hormone (GnRH) Agonists

−Gonadotropin Releasing Hormone (GnRH) Antagonists

Treatment of Polycystic Ovarian Syndrome (PCOS)

Weight loss for obese women is important, not only for improving chances of ovulation, but also for reducing the risks during pregnancy.

CC is the first-line drug for treatment of anovulation.

Metformin is an insulin-sensitizing agent that has been used with off-label indication in the treatment of PCOS.

Gonadotropin therapy for ovulation induction in women with PCOS has been shown to be successful with pregnancy rates of approximately 22%.

Ovarian drilling involves drilling 3 to 10 holes per ovary at laparoscopy using electrocautery or laser.

Risks of the surgery include ovarian adhesions and ovarian failure if too many holes are drilled.

Treatment of Prolactinomas

Medical therapy involves the use of dopamine agonists to suppress prolactin secretion.

The most commonly used dopamine agonist is bromocriptine.

Cabergoline is a newer option and has fewer side effects.

Once the prolactin level is normalized, ovulation will be restored within a few months.

Macroadenomas can be treated medically, but surgery is often the preferred method for large masses.

FALLOPIAN TUBES

The fallopian tubes (also referred to as uterine tubes or oviducts) are uterine appendages located bilaterally at the superior portion of the cavity.

The fallopian tubes exit the uterus through an area known as the cornua and form a connection between the endometrial and peritoneal cavities.

Each tube is approximately 10 cm in length and 1 cm in diameter and is situated within a portion of the broad ligament called the mesosalpinx.

The distal portion of the fallopian tube ends in an orientation encircling the ovary.

The fallopian tube has 4 parts.

– The first segment, closest to the uterus, is called the isthmus.

– The second segment is the ampulla, which becomes more dilated in diameter and is the typical place of fertilization.

– The final segment, furthest from the uterus, is the infundibulum.

– The infundibulum gives rise to the fimbriae, fingerlike projections that are responsible for catching the egg that is released by the ovary.

The arterial supply to the fallopian tubes is from branches of the uterine and ovarian arteries, located within the mesosalpinx.

Lymphatic drainage of the fallopian tubes is through the iliac and aortic nodes.

The nerve supply to the fallopian tubes is via both sympathetic and parasympathetic fibers; sensory fibers run from thoracic segments 11-12 and lumbar segment 1.

Microscopic Anatomy

The tubal mucosa has many folds, or plicae, which are most evident in the ampulla; a smooth muscular layer surrounds the mucosa.

Within the mucosa of the uterine tubes, 3 different cell types exist:

– Columnar ciliated epithelial cells (25%).

– Secretory cells (60%).

– Narrow peg cells (< 10%).

Functions

The released (ovulated) oocyte is guided by waving movements of the infundibulum and fimbriae; muscular peristalsis moves the egg through the fallopian tube.

Fertilization usually occurs in the distal third of the fallopian tube adjacent to ovary (ampulla).

Peristalsis moves the fertilized oocyte through the tubal isthmus and into the uterus for implantation.

Estradiol promotes growth, proliferation and ciliogenesis.

Both estradiol and progesterone increase contractions of the muscular layer to promote transport of the oocyte and fertilized zygote.

The composition of the oviductal fluid is crucial to the survival and development of the zygote; it is tightly regulated by the secretory epithelial cells.

The fluid is enriched in sodium and potassium; oviductal fluid also is enriched in lactic acid and bicarbonate, which are important for cleavage of fertilized eggs or zygotes.

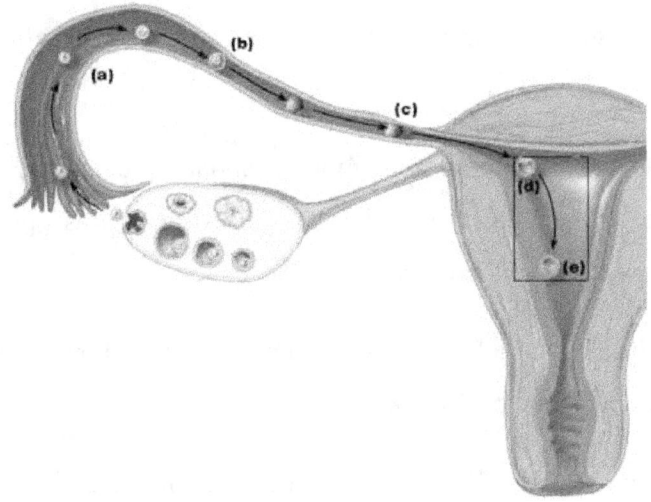

Fallopian (Uterine) Tubes

FERTILIZATION

The fallopian tubes, or oviducts, function as conduits for the oocyte and spermatozoa, and they provide nutrients for the gametes and early embryo, as well as serving as the site of fertilization.

Ciliated cells at the open, fimbriated end (ostium) direct the oocyte into the infundibulum and down through the ampulla.

Fertilization usually occurs in the distal third of the fallopian tube adjacent to ovary (ampulla).

The zygote is kept in the fallopian tube for about three days by the spastic contractions of the estrogen-dominated isthmus; as progesterone increases, muscle tone decreases.

Oviductal fluid is enriched in lactic acid and bicarbonate, which are important for cleavage of fertilized eggs or zygotes.

Once the zygote divides it is called an embryo; while still in the fallopian tube, the embryo undergoes cleavage division (1-cell to 8-cell), compaction and blastocyst formation before it reaches the uterus.

The inner cell mass of the embryo becomes the fetus and the outer cells become the placenta and fetal membranes.

Peristalsis moves the fertilized oocyte through the tubal isthmus and into the uterus for implantation.

Approximately seven days after fertilization, the blastocyst bursts from the zona pellucida (hatching) and implants in the wall of the uterus.

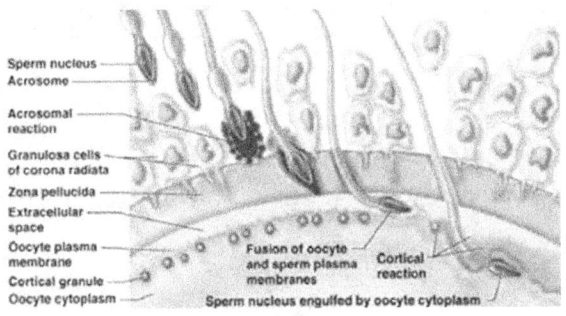

Fertilization

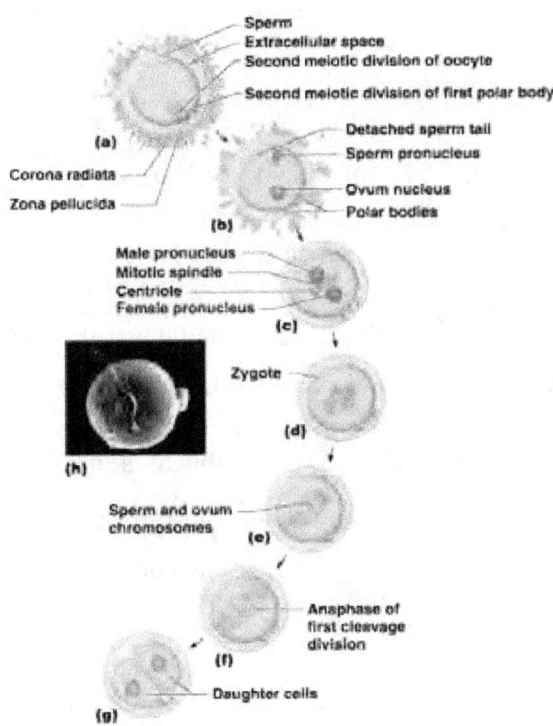

Embryo Cleavage

TUBAL FACTORS OF INFERTILITY

Causes

Abnormalities or damage to the fallopian tube interferes with fertility and is responsible for abnormal implantation (eg, ectopic pregnancy).

Obstruction of the distal end of the fallopian tubes results in accumulation of the normally secreted tubal fluid, creating distention of the tube with subsequent damage of the epithelial cilia (hydrosalpinx).

Other tubal factors associated with infertility are either congenital or acquired.

Congenital absence of the fallopian tubes can be due to spontaneous torsion in utero followed by necrosis and reabsorption.

Elective tubal ligation and salpingectomy are acquired causes.

Anatomical defects or physiologic dysfunctions of the peritoneal cavity, including infection, adhesions, and adnexal masses, may cause infertility.

Pelvic inflammatory disease (PID), peritoneal adhesions secondary to previous pelvic surgery, endometriosis, and ovarian cyst rupture all compromise the motility of the fallopian tubes or produce blockage of the fimbriae with development of hydrosalpinx.

Large myomas, pelvic masses, or blockage of the cul-de-sac interferes interferes with the normal oocyte pickup mechanism.

Peri-ovarian adhesions interfere with the normal oocyte release at ovulation, becoming a mechanical factor for infertility.

Investigations

Hysterosalpingogram (HSG) and laparoscopy.

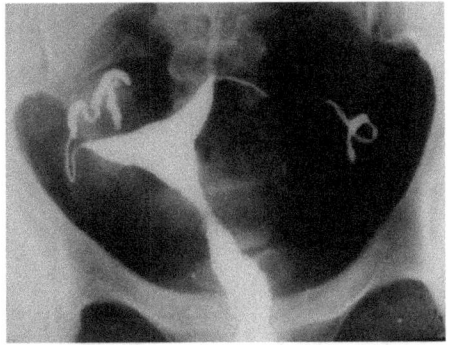 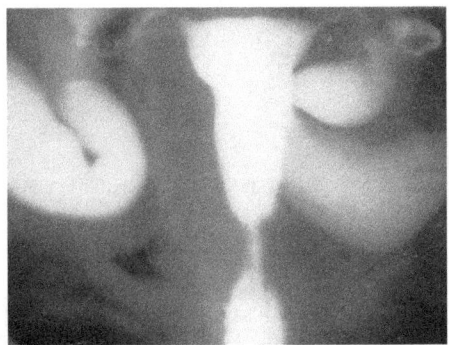

          Normal   **Hydrosalpinx**

Hysterosalpingogram (HSG)

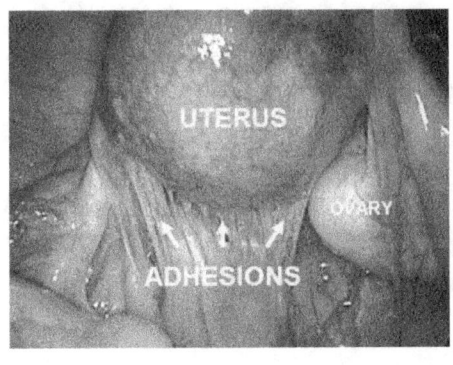 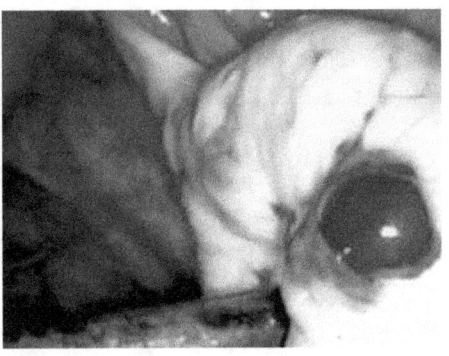

   Pelvic Adhesions   **Ovarian Endometriosis**

Laparoscopy

Treatment

Tubal reconstruction was the only hope for those patients before assisted reproductive therapy became available.

Tubal Surgery

Tubal obstruction and adhesions can be corrected through laparotomy, operative laparoscopy, and, in special circumstances, through operative hysteroscopy and tubal cannulation.

Lysis of adhesions should be meticulous, using hydrodissection and fine instruments.

Treatment of hydrosalpinx (distal tubal obstruction) with salpingostomy can be performed through microsurgery or operative laparoscopy.

If the fallopian tubes are beyond repair, bilateral salpingectomy with destruction of the cornual area is recommended in preparation for IVF.

Assisted Reproduction Techniques (ART)

ART used to treat infertility include the following:

– Intrauterine insemination (IUI).

– In vitro fertilization (IVF).

– Gamete intrafallopian transfer (GIFT).

– Zygote intrafallopian transfer (ZIFT).

– Intracytoplasmic sperm injection (ICSI).

Treatment of Endometriosis

Endometriosis treatment may be divided according to the severity of the disease and patient needs.

Four alternatives are currently available to treat endometriosis:

- Expectant therapy should be based on a complete workup with diagnosis of very early stages of the disease (minimal) in patients without clinical symptoms, ie, an incidental finding.

- Surgical treatment should be directed at destroying the disease using electrocoagulation, laser vaporization, endocoagulation, or excision.

- Medical treatment is directed toward suppressing estrogen production by the ovary with oral contraceptives, progestins, androgens (eg, danazol), or GnRH agonists (eg, Leuprolide acetate).

- Combined medical and surgical treatments are usually used for the treatment of severe endometriosis.

UTERUS

The uterus is the inverted pear-shaped female reproductive organ that lies in the midline of the body, within the pelvis between the bladder and the rectum.

It is thick-walled and muscular, with a lining that, during reproductive years, changes in response to hormone stimulation throughout a woman's monthly cycle.

The uterus can be divided into 3 parts:

– The most inferior aspect is the cervix, and

– The bulk of the organ is called the body of the uterus (corpus uteri).

– Between these 2 is the isthmus, a short area of constriction.

The body of the uterus is globe-shaped and is typically situated in an anteverted position, at a 90° angle to the vagina.

The upper aspect of the body is dome-shaped and is called the fundus; it is typically the most muscular part of the uterus.

The body of the uterus is responsible for holding a pregnancy, and strong uterine wall contractions help to expel the fetus during labor and delivery.

The average weight of a nonpregnant, nulliparous uterus is approximately 40-50 g.

A multiparous uterus may weigh slightly more than this, with an upper limit of approximately 110 g.

A menopausal uterus is small and atrophied and typically weighs much less.

The uterine cavity is flattened and triangular; the uterine tubes enter the cavity bilaterally in the superolateral portion of the cavity.

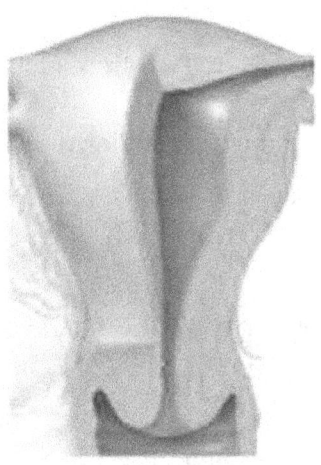

Uterine Cavity

The uterus is connected to its surrounding structures by a series of ligaments and connective tissue.

The pelvic peritoneum is attached to the body and the cervix as the broad ligament, reflecting onto the bladder, and attaches the uterus to the lateral pelvic side walls.

Within the broad base of the broad ligament, connective tissue strands associated with the uterine and vaginal vessels help to support the uterus and vagina; together, these strands are referred to as cardinal ligament.

Rectouterine ligaments, lying within peritoneal folds, stretch posteriorly from the cervix to reach the sacrum.

The round ligaments of the uterus are much denser structures and connect the uterus to the anterolateral abdominal wall at the deep inguinal ring; they lie within the anterior lamina of the broad ligament.

Within the round ligament is the artery of Sampson, a small artery that must be ligated during hysterectomy.

The vasculature of the uterus is derived from uterine arteries and veins.

The uterine vessels arise from the anterior division of the internal iliac, and branches of the uterine artery anastomose with the ovarian artery along the uterine tube.

Lymphatic drainage is primarily to the lateral aortic, pelvic, and iliac nodes that surround the iliac vessels.

The nerve supply is attained through

– The sympathetic nervous system (by way of the hypogastric and ovarian plexuses) and

– The parasympathetic nervous system (by way of the pelvic splanchnic nerves from the second through fourth sacral nerves).

Microscopic Anatomy

The uterine corpus has 3 layers, from outermost to innermost:

– The serosa is a continuation of the visceral peritoneum.

– The myometrium is composed of 3 layers of smooth muscle.

– The endometrium is composed of of 2 layers:

(1) The basal layer lies next to the myometrium and contains stem cells, blood vessels and glands; it builds the functional layer in response to changing levels of estrogens and progesterone produced in the ovary and secreted into the blood stream.

(2) The functional layer contains blood vessels and glands.

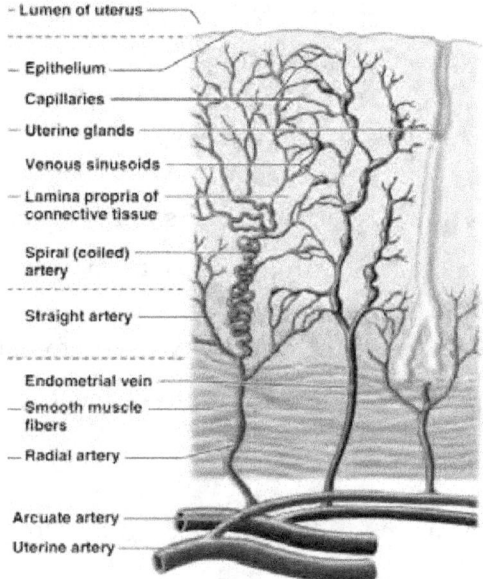

Endometrium

Functions

It contains and nourishes the embryo and fetus from the time the fertilized egg is implanted to the time of birth of the fetus.

ENDOMETRIAL CYCLE

Proliferative Phase

The preovulatory follicular phase begins with menses; FSH and LH are released with each GnRH pulse.

Inhibin secretion is low so that FSH, which began to rise late in the luteal phase of the prior cycle, continues to rise.

At the same time, LH levels start to rise slowly.

Several secondary follicles of different sizes are recruited, and they secrete increasing amounts of estrogen and inhibin.

Estrogen and IGF-I increase the sensitivity of the follicle to FSH, while inhibin blunts the pituitary FSH response to GnRH leading to a decrease in plasma FSH.

The follicle most sensitive to FSH continues to develop and becomes the dominant follicle.

Less developed, that is, less sensitive, follicles undergo degeneration (atresia) because of insufficient FSH.

Estrogen decreases the amplitude of GnRH pulses, as well as increases pituitary sensitivity to GnRH.

Estrogen causes proliferation and vascularization of the endometrium, and increases myometrial contractility.

Estrogen also causes the cervical mucus to become clear and thin.

Secretory Phase

When plasma estradiol exceeds 150-200 pg/mL for 36 hours, GnRH triggers a large surge of LH and a small surge of FSH.

The FSH surge recruits new follicles for the next cycle; the LH surge triggers ovulation and luteinization of follicular cells.

The corpus luteum then synthesizes increasing amounts of progesterone, estradiol, and inhibin.

FSH and LH are low, but they maintain the corpus luteum.

Progesterone decreases the frequency of GnRH pulses resulting in a decrease in the frequency of LH pulses.

The LH pulse amplitude increases, however, so that plasma LH remains unchanged.

The post-ovulatory rise in progesterone appears to be responsible for the rise in basal body temperature.

Progesterone decreases myometrial excitability and increases endometrial secretory activity.

The luteal phase has a more constant length than the follicular phase.

Menstrual Phase

If implantation of the blastocyst occurs, the lifespan of the corpus luteum is prolonged by hCG, which is produced by the developing embryo.

If implantation does not occur, the corpus luteum regresses.

Luteal regression begins 14-15 days after ovulation, and progesterone levels decrease to follicular phase levels.

The endometrial lining undergoes ischemic necrosis followed by menses, which is desquamation and bleeding.

Menstruation lasts 3-5 days, and on average, 35 ml of blood + 35 ml serous fluid are lost.

One day before menstruation, when the inhibin levels are low, FSH begins to rise - the proliferative phase is again initiated.

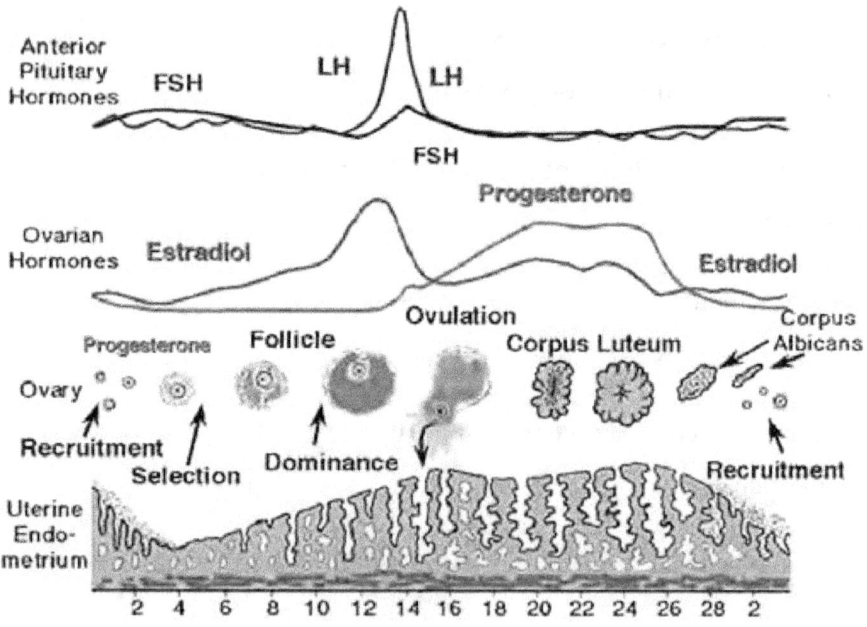

Endometrial Cycle

IMPLANTATION

Approximately seven days after fertilization, the blastocyst bursts from the zona pellucida (hatching) and implants in the wall of the uterus.

Implantation requires prior conditioning of the endometrium by progesterone, which causes the stromal cells to swell and accumulate glycogen, lipids and protein.

The presence of hCG from the blastocyst stimulates the corpus luteum of the maternal ovary to secrete progesterone.

The blastocyst attaches to the uterine fundus at the embryonic pole.

Trophoblast cells then invade through the endometrial epithelium into the endometrial stroma aided by proteases.

Stromal cells decidualize; a process by which they enlarge and become transcriptionally active, and surround the blastocyst.

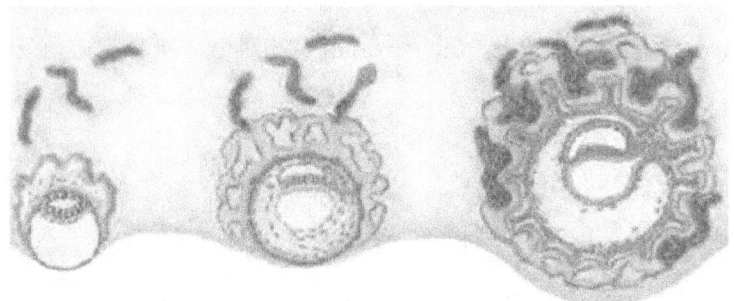

Implantation

EMBRYO DEVELOPMENT

The zygote is kept in the fallopian tube for about three days by the spastic contractions of the estrogen-dominated isthmus; as progesterone increases, muscle tone decreases.

In the fallopian tube, the zygote undergoes cleavage division (1-cell to 8-cell), compaction and blastocyst formation.

The inner cell mass becomes the fetus and the outer cells become the placenta and fetal membranes.

Peristalsis moves the fertilized oocyte through the tubal isthmus and into the uterus for implantation.

Approximately seven days after fertilization, the blastocyst bursts from the zona pellucida, which is called hatching, and implants in the wall of the uterus, which is called nidation.

Implantation requires prior conditioning of the endometrium by progesterone, which causes the stromal cells to swell and accumulate glycogen, lipids and protein.

The presence of hCG from the blastocyst stimulates the corpus luteum of the maternal ovary to secrete progesterone.

The blastocyst attaches to the wall of the uterine fundus at the embryonic pole.

Trophoblast cells then invade through the endometrial epithelium into the endometrial stroma aided by proteases.

Stromal cells decidualize; a process by which they enlarge and become transcriptionally active, and surround the blastocyst.

Within 11 days of fertilization, the trophoblast forms two layers, the cytotrophoblast and the syncytiotrophoblast, containing lacunae.

The placenta forms a barrier to permit exchange of nutrients, gases and wastes with only slight mixing of fetal blood with maternal blood.

Fetal blood cells can normally be found in the maternal circulation in all cases.

As the lacunae enlarge, the trophoblast forms villi, which consist of a vascularized core of cytotrophoblast covered by syncytiotrophoblast.

The trophoblast erodes the maternal spiral arteries, which then flow directly into the intervillous spaces.

The fully developed placenta consists of the following three layers of membranes:

– Amnion (inner), which is a single layer of ectodermal epithelium completely enclosing the embryo;

– Chorion (outer), which surrounds the amniotic sac and includes the villi and trophoblast; and

– The decidua of the maternal endometrium.

The uterofetoplacental circulation is established by about 6 gestational weeks and is completed by 10 weeks, connecting the maternal decidua through the chorionic villi to the fetus via the umbilical vessels.

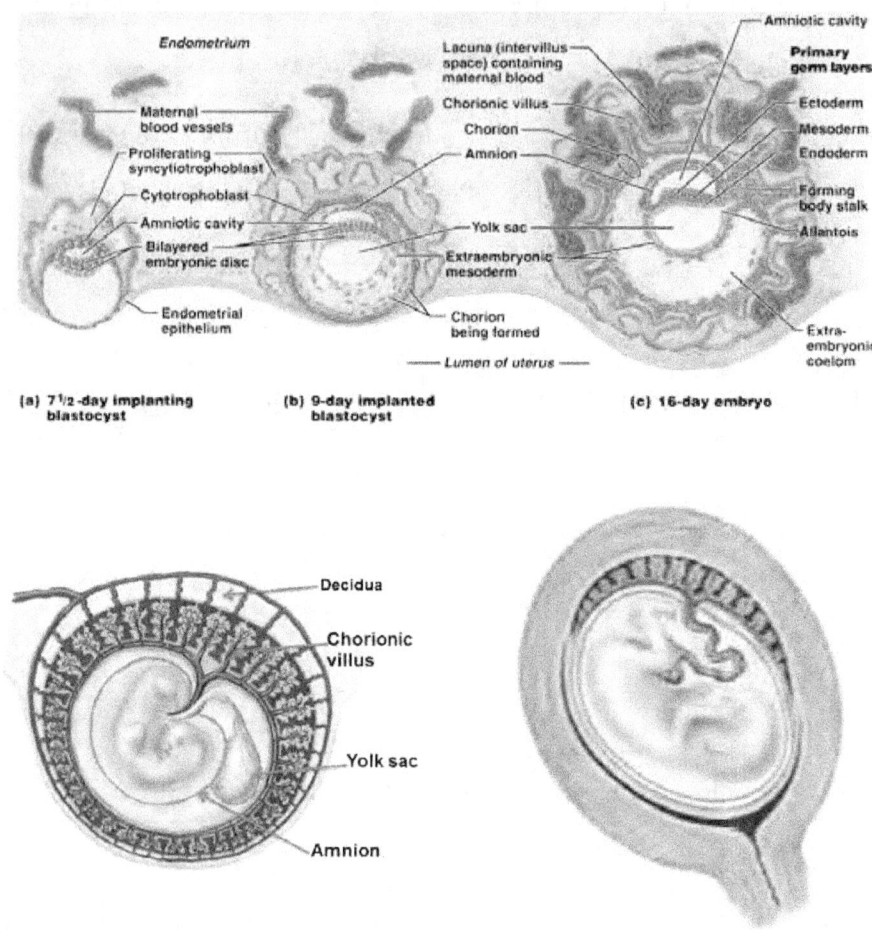

Embryo Development

UTERINE FACTORS OF INFERTILITY

Causes

Uterine factors can be congenital or acquired.

The full spectrum of congenital/müllerian abnormalities varies from total absence of the uterus and vagina (Rokitansky-Küster-Hauser syndrome) to minor defects such as arcuate uterus and vaginal septa (transverse or longitudinal).

The relationship between müllerian anomalies and infertility is not entirely clear except when absolute absence of the uterus, cervix, vagina, or a combination of these occurs.

Premature delivery has been associated with cervical incompetence, unicornuate uterus associated with a blind horn, and septate uterus.

Septate uterus may also be responsible for implantation problems and first-trimester miscarriages.

Endometritis associated with a traumatic delivery, dilatation and curettage, intrauterine device, or any instrumentation (eg, myomectomy, hysteroscopy) of the endometrial cavity may create intrauterine adhesions, with partial or total obliteration of the uterineendometrial cavity.

Intrauterine and submucosal fibroids may be implicated in implantation failure, early miscarriages, premature delivery, and abruptio placentae.

Investigations

Hysterosalpingogram (HSG) - most frequently used to assess endometrial cavity; pelvic ultrasonogram; saline infusion sonogram (SIS); pelvic magnetic resonance imaging; hysteroscopy; and endometrial biopsy.

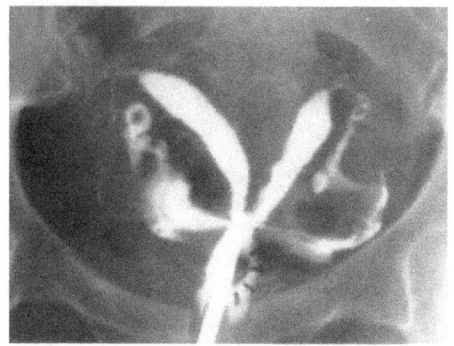
Septate Uterus

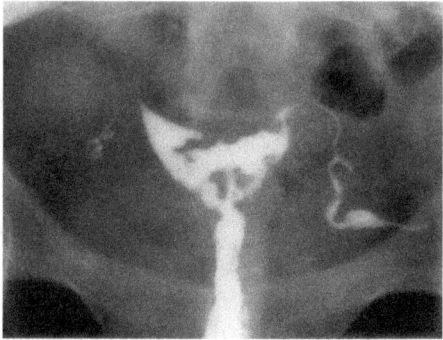
Endometrial Polyps

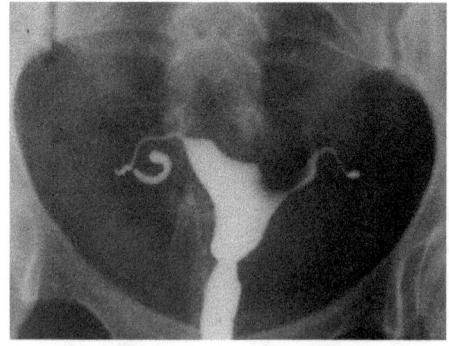
Submucous Fibroid

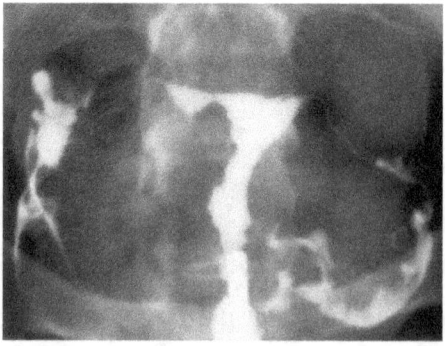
Intrauterine Adhesions

Hysterosalpingogram (HSG)

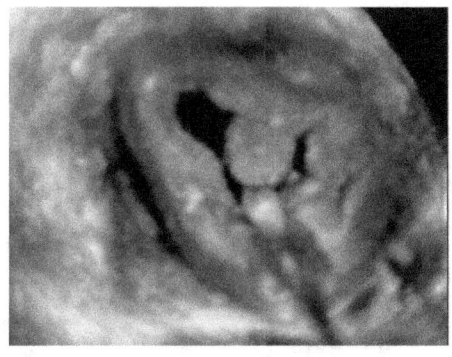 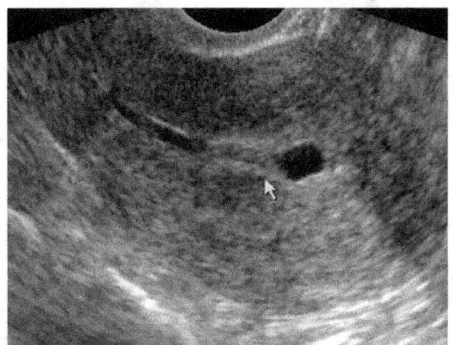

Submucous Fibroid **Intrauterine Adhesions**

Saline Infusion Sonography (SIS)

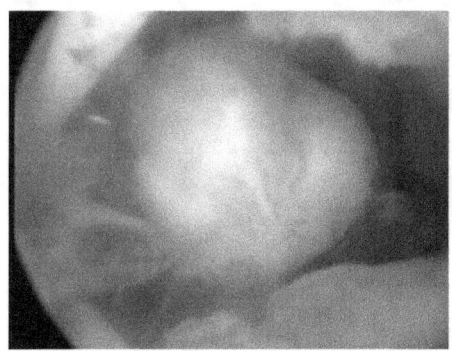 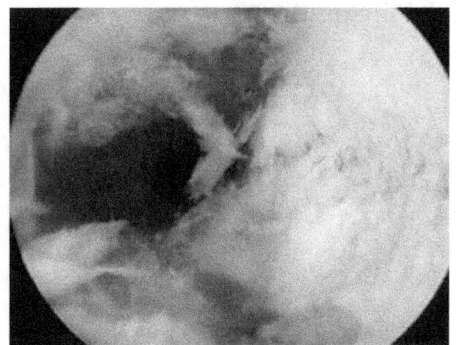

Submucous Fibroid **Intrauterine Adhesions**

Hysteroscopy

Treatment

Surgical management of uterine factor infertility includes laparotomy, laparoscopy, or hysteroscopy.

Septate Uterus

Uterine anomalies can be corrected through operative hysteroscopy under general anesthesia or conscious sedation.

Uterine Synechiae

Uterine synechiae are corrected using operative hysteroscopy; in many instances, more than one hysteroscopy is required.

Endometrial Polyps

Endometrial polyps are removed through operative hysteroscopy associated with a dilatation and curettage, if necessary.

Uterine Fibroids

- Medical treatment is a temporary treatment, ideally used for patients who are close to menopause or who are risky surgical candidates.

- Surgical treatment of myomas includes conventional laparotomy, operative laparoscopy, and operative hysteroscopy.

- Uterine fibroid embolization consists of catheterization of the uterine artery and the injection of microbeads of polyvinyl alcohol to selectively occlude the circulation of the fibroid.

CERVIX

The cervix is the inferior portion of the uterus, separating the body of the uterus from the vagina; its average length is 3-5 cm.

The cervix is cylindrical in shape, with an endocervical canal located in the midline, allowing passage of semen into the uterus.

The external opening into the vagina is termed the external os; and the internal opening into the endometrial cavity is termed the internal os.

The internal os is the portion of a female cervix that dilates to allow delivery of the fetus during labor.

The vasculature is supplied by descending branches of the uterine artery, which run bilaterally at the 3 o'clock and 9 o'clock position of the cervix.

Lymphatic drainage of the cervix is complex: the obturator, common iliac, internal iliac, external iliac, and visceral parametrial nodes are the main drainage points.

The nerve supply to the cervix is via the parasympathetic nervous system by way of the second through fourth sacral segments; many pain nerve fibers run alongside these parasympathetics.

Microscopic Anatomy

Most of the cervix is composed of collagenous connective tissue, smooth muscle, and mucopolysaccharide ground substance.

The endocervical canal is rich in mucous glands and is primarily columnar epithelium.

The external portion of the cervix that lies within the vagina is composed of stratified squamous epithelium.

The area surrounding the external os is termed the transformation zone, which is the transition point between squamous cells externally and columnar cells of the endocervical canal.

Functions

The epithelial lining, of the cervix consists of tall, secretory columnar cells that respond to estradiol by increasing in height and accumulating cervical mucus rich in protein substances.

The mucus functions as a hormone-dependent barrier for sperm to enter the uterus.

At mid-cycle, when estrogen levels are high, mucus is clear, thin, and copious with high elasticity, called spinnbarkeit.

At this point, the cervical mucus is permeable to sperm and when dried, has a characteristic microscopic ferning appearance.

The mucus actually restricts sperm with poor morphology and motility; as a result, only a minority of ejaculated sperm actually enters the cervix.

In response to progesterone production after ovulation, mucus production decreases and it becomes viscous, cloudy, and impermeable to sperm.

CAPACITATION

After the ejaculation, the sperm cells go through several essential physiological changes during their time in the female genital tract before they, at the end, are able to penetrate the oocyte membrane.

The first change in this cascade is capacitation, which is physiological maturation process of the sperm cell membranes.

The sperm cells accomplish this during the ascension through the female genital tract (in contact with its secretions); the cervix may act as a site where capacitation of the sperm might start.

The changes take place via the sperm cell membrane in which it may be that receptors are made available through removal of a glycoprotein layer.

The area of the acrosomal cap is also so altered thereby that the acrosome reaction becomes possible.

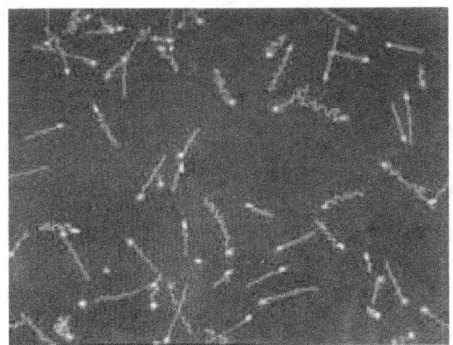 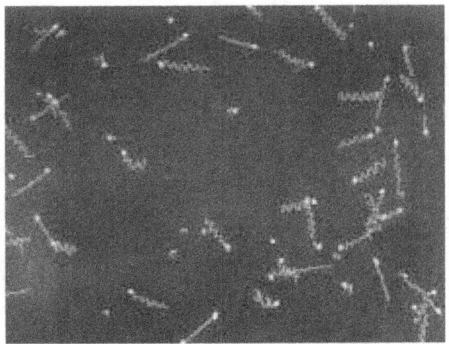

Before Capacitation **After Capacitation**

CERVICAL FACTORS OF INFERTILITY

Causes

Cervical factor infertility can be caused by stenosis or abnormalities of the mucus-sperm interaction.

Cervical stenosis can be congenital or acquired in etiology, resulting from surgical procedures, infections, hypoestrogenism, and radiation therapy.

Mucus secretion may be altered by hormonal changes and medications, especially drugs like CC, which decrease the production.

Investigations

Cervical stenosis can be diagnosed during a speculum examination.

The postcoital test (PCT) consists of evaluating the amount of spermatozoa and its motility within the cervical mucus during the preovulatory period.

Treatment

Chronic cervicitis may be treated with antibiotics.

Reduced secretion of cervical mucus due to destruction of the endocervical glands by previous cervical conization, freezing, or laser vaporization responds poorly to low-dose estrogen therapy.

The easiest and most successful treatment is IUI.

MALE REPRODUCTIVE BIOLOGY

The male reproductive system is a network of external and internal organs that has two major functions:

– Produce and deliver spermatozoa, for sexual reproduction.

– Produce hormones that regulate reproductive function and secondary sex characteristics.

Sperm produced in the testes is transported through the epididymis, ductus deferens, ejaculatory duct, and urethra.

The seminal vesicles, prostate gland, and bulbourethral gland produce seminal fluid that accompany and nourish the sperm as it is emitted from the penis during ejaculation and throughout the fertilization process.

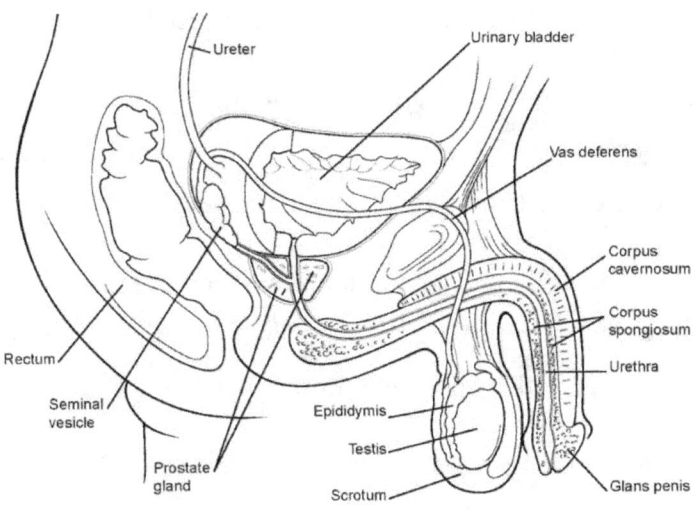

Male Reproductive System

HORMONAL CONTROL

– GnRH is secreted by the hypothalamus and stimulates the pituitary to synthesize and release LH and FSH.

– LH stimulates Leydig cells to synthesize testosterone.

– FSH maintains Sertoli cell function.

Testosterone

Testosterone has significant reproductive and nonreproductive effects throughout the male life cycle.

Before birth, testosterone masculinizes the reproductive tract and external genitalia and promotes descent of the testes into the scrotum.

For sex-specific tissues, testosterone promotes growth and maturation of the reproductive system at puberty, is essential for spermatogenesis, and maintains the reproductive tract throughout adulthood.

Other reproductive effects include development of the sex drive at puberty and control of gonadotropin hormone secretion; secondary sex characteristics are also testosterone-dependent.

Testosterone induces the male pattern of hair growth (such as the beard), causes the voice to deepen due to thickening of the vocal cords, and promotes muscle growth responsible for the male body configuration.

Nonreproductive actions of testosterone include a protein anabolic effect, promotion of bone growth at puberty and closure of the epiphyseal plates.

Pituitary Feedback

Testosterone provides negative feedback to the pituitary to decrease LH and FSH levels, and to the hypothalamus to decrease GnRH production.

Inhibin, produced by Sertoli cells, is responsible for the remainder of the inhibition of FSH production.

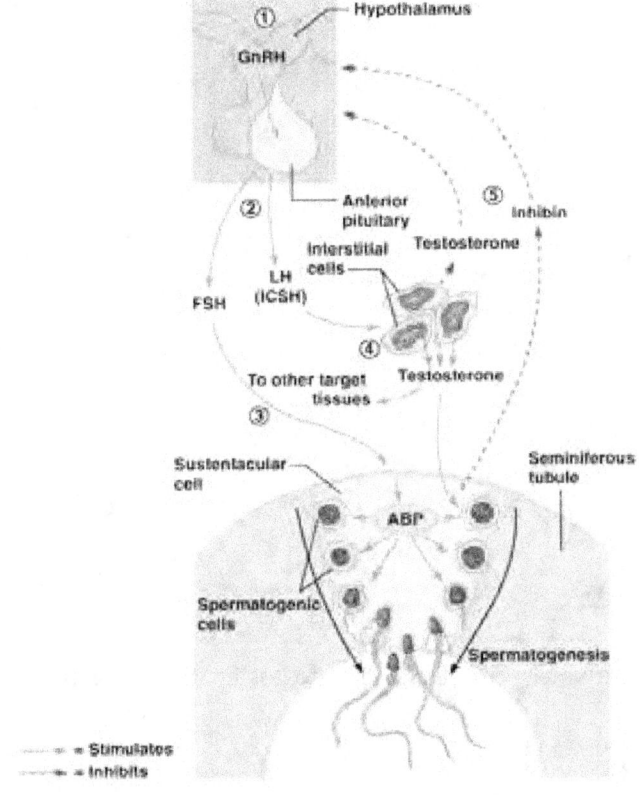

Hormonal Control of Testicular Function

PRETESTICULAR FACTORS OF INFERTILITY

Causes

Pretesticular causes of infertility include congenital or acquired diseases of the hypothalamus, pituitary, or peripheral organs that alter the hypothalamic-pituitary axis leading to hypogonadotropic hypogonadism.

− Laurence-Moon-Biedl syndrome.

− Kallmann syndrome.

− Prolactinoma.

− Isolated LH deficiency.

− Isolated FSH deficiency.

− Cushing disease.

− Congenital Adrenal Hyperplasia (CAH)

Investigations

− Hormonal analysis (FSH, LH, TSH, testosterone, prolactin).

− Skull X-ray, CT, MRI.

Treatment

− Treatment of endocrinopathies.

− Sperm retrieval techniques (MESA, PESA, TESE) / ICSI.

TESTES

The testes are the primary male reproductive organ and are responsible for testosterone and sperm production.

Their development is influenced by the presence of the Y sex chromosome and by maternal hormonal levels.

The testes develop in the fetal abdomen and begin descent during the 7th month of pregnancy.

The male sex organs are formed under the influence of testosterone secreted from the fetal testes.

Failure to descend, called cryptorchidism, results in sterility, which is a lack of spermatozoa, and, frequently, abnormally low testosterone.

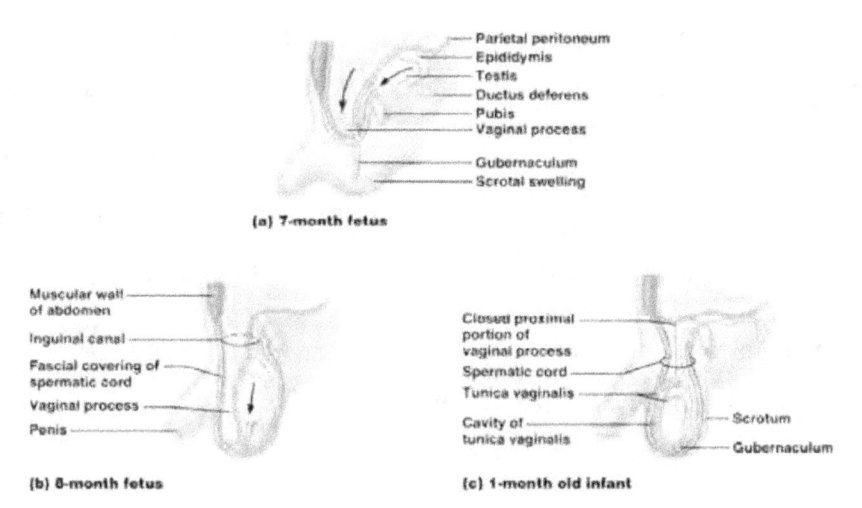

Testicular Descend

Each testis is 4-5 cm long, 2-3 cm wide, weighs 10-14 g and is suspended in the scrotum by the dartos muscle and spermatic cord.

Suspension outside the body cavity permits spermatogenesis at 36°C.

Each testis is covered by the tunica vaginalis testis, tunica albuginea, and tunica vasculosa.

The tunica vaginalis testis is the lower portion of the processus vaginalis and is reflected from the testes on the inner surface of the scrotum, thus forming the visceral and parietal layers.

Beneath the visceral layer of the tunica vaginalis is the tunica albuginea, which forms a dense covering for the testes.

Internal to the tunica albuginea is the tunica vasculosa, containing a plexus of blood vessels and connective tissue.

Bilateral testicular arteries originating from the aorta, just inferior to the renal arteries, enter the scrotum in the spermatic cord via the inguinal canal, and split into two branches at the posterosuperior border of the testis.

Additionally, the testes receive blood from the cremasteric branch of the inferior epigastric artery and the artery to the ductus deferens.

The pampiniform plexus drains both the testis and epididymis before coalescing to form the testicular vein, usually above the spermatic cord formation at the deep inguinal ring.

Lymphatic drainage via the testicular vessels passes into the abdomen, ending in the lateral aortic and pre-aortic nodes.

The tenth and eleventh thoracic spinal nerves supply the testes via the renal and aortic autonomic plexuses.

Microscopic Anatomy

The testes are divided into approximately 400 segments called lobules each of which is occupied by 2-4 seminiferous tubules, which are responsible for producing spermatozoa.

Each testis has 600-1200 seminiferous tubules with a total length of 280-400-m.

At the mediastinum testis, on the posterior border of the testis, the seminiferous tubules empty spermatozoa into the tubuli recti and rete testis, eventually coalescing to form 6-8 efferent ductules draining spermatozoa into the epididymis.

The seminiferous tubule epithelium consists of proliferating spermatogenic cells and the sustentacular Sertoli cells.

Spermatogenic cells are at various stages of spermatogenesis and Sertoli cells are columnar cells that extend from the basement membrane to the lumen of the seminiferous tubule.

Interstitial cells in the testis, including the Leydig cells, constitute 20-30% of the tissue in the gland and are found in between seminiferous tubules.

The washed out cytoplasm of the Leydig cells is due high lipid content in the form of cholesterol for synthesis of testosterone.

The seminiferous tubules are the site of spermatogenesis; there are approximately 244 m (800 feet) of seminiferous tubules in each testis.

Each tubule consists of a basement membrane, lined with germ cells that become spermatozoa, and Sertoli cells; these tubules increase in diameter and tortuosity with hormonal changes of puberty.

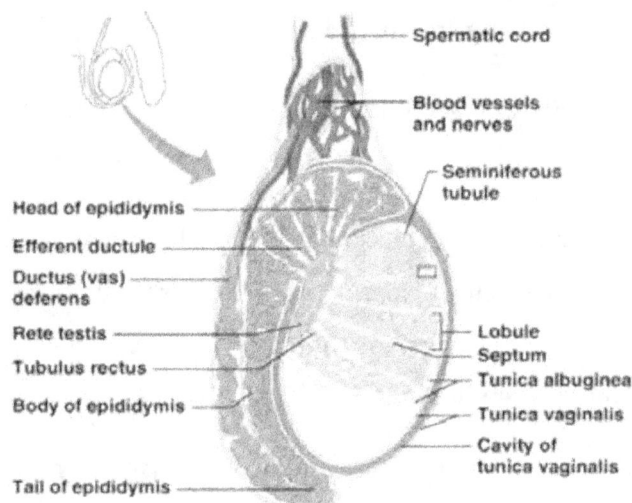

Seminiferous Tubules

There are three unique cell types within the testes:

– Germ cells, the cells that divide and mature to become sperm.

– Sertoli cells, which provide crucial support for spermatogenesis.

– Leydig cells that produce the androgenic hormone testosterone, which maintains the reproductive tract and secondary sex characteristics.

All germ cells and Sertoli cells are within the seminiferous tubule, while Leydig cells are outside the tubules.

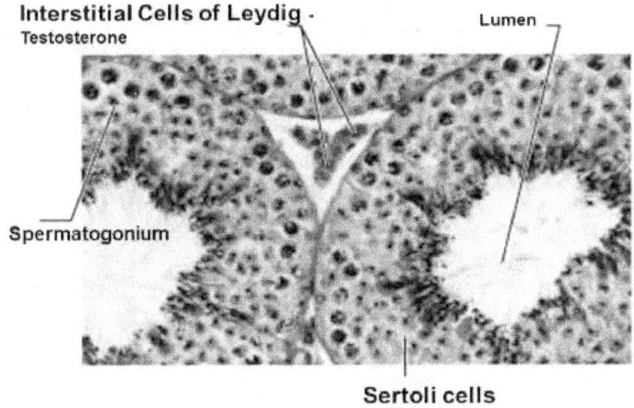

Cell Types within the Testes

Functions

– Produce germ cells (spermatozoa) for sexual reproduction.

– Produce testosterone that regulates reproductive function and secondary sex characteristics.

SPERMATOGENESIS

Beginning at puberty, spermatogenesis occurs continuously and repeatedly within folds of the Sertoli cells.

Spermatogonia (the sperm stem cells) lie at the base of the Sertoli cells and proliferate through mitosis to produce daughter cells that enter spermatogenesis.

In the two-step reduction division process of meiosis, spermatocytes and spermatids develop; spermatids are haploid, containing only one copy of each chromosome.

As the germ cells divide and mature, they move away from the base of the tubule toward the apical surface of Sertoli cells.

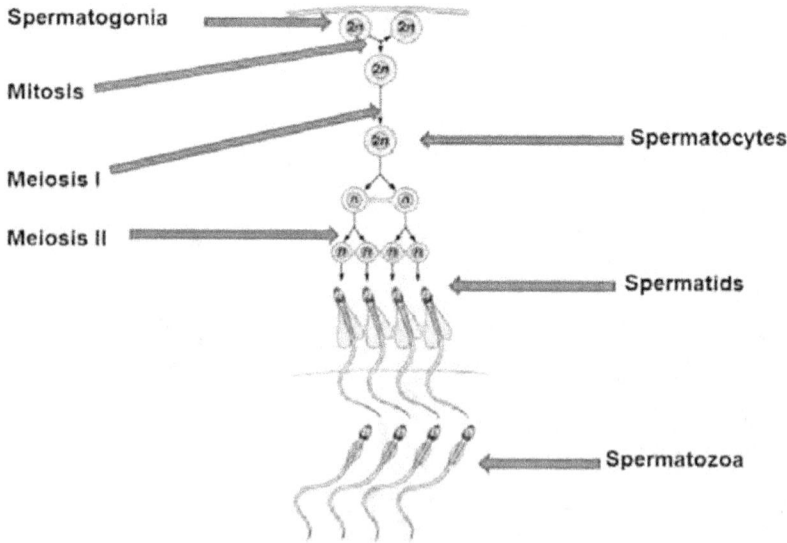

Spermatogenesis

Spermiogenesis

Following meiosis, spermiogenesis is the maturation process in which the round spermatids are transformed into elongated spermatozoa with tails.

The spermatid nucleus condenses and most cytoplasm is lost; the Golgi apparatus moves to one side of the nucleus, forming an acrosome that surrounds the top two thirds of the nucleus (in the head).

Cell microtubules organize into a flagellar apparatus to form the tail for motility, and mitochondria for movement.

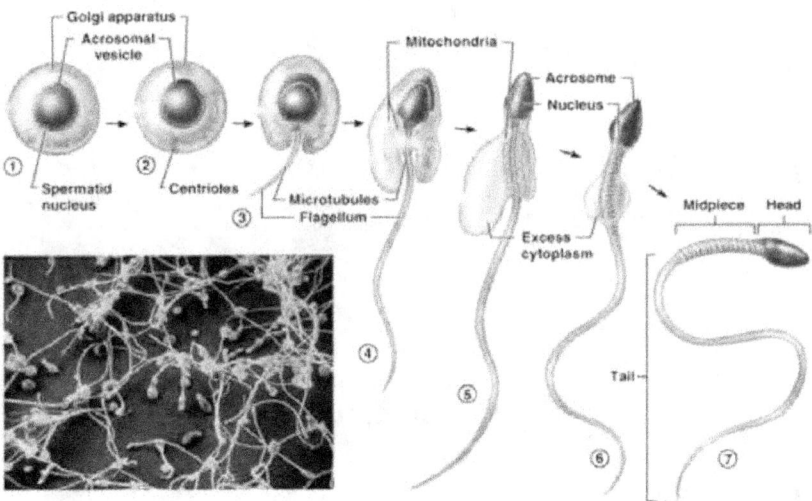

Spermiogenesis

Spermiation

Spermiation is the process in which fully developed but non-motile spermatozoa are released from the Sertoli cells and propelled out of the tubules into the collecting tubules, rete testis and then the epididymis.

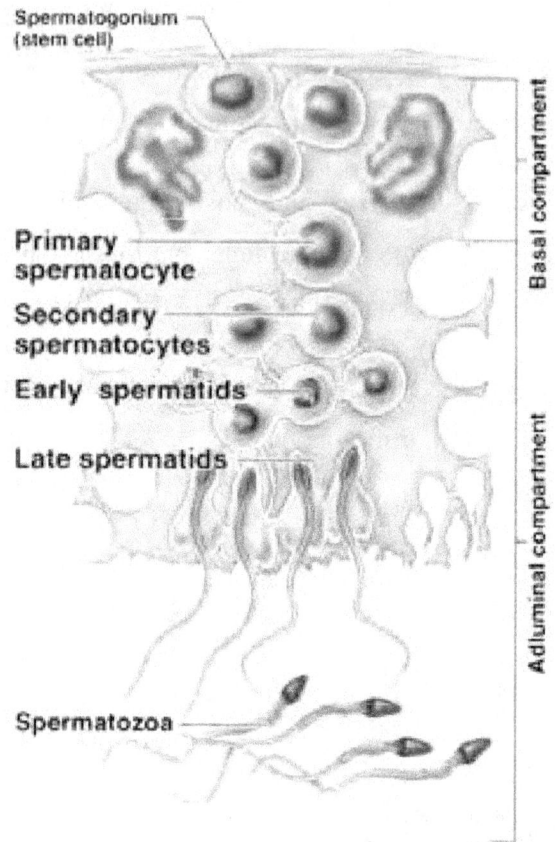

Spermiation

Mature Sperm

Mature sperm have a head, which consists primarily of the nucleus containing genetic information.

The acrosome is a specialized lysosome, containing about 20 different enzymes, which are needed for penetration of the ovum during fertilization.

The acrosome covers the anterior third of the nucleus in a mature sperm.

In the midpiece are mitochondria to provide the energy required for the movement of the tail.

The tail grows out of one of the centrioles; movement results from the sliding of the microtubules.

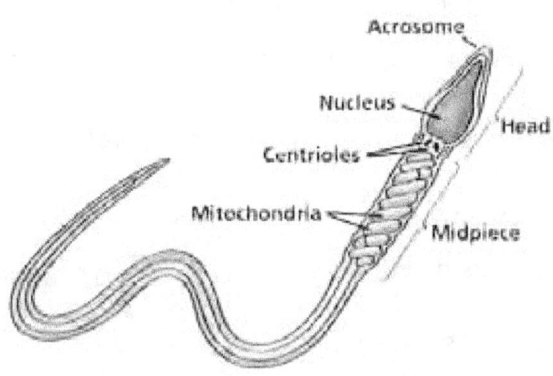

Mature Sperm

Normal Sperm Morphology

Normal sperm morphology is defined by multiple parameters:

– The head is oval shaped, 4-5 microns long, 2-3 microns wide, the length-to-width ratio is 1.5 to 1.75, and a well-defined acrosome makes up 40 to 70% of the head area.

– The midpiece is intact and there is no cytoplasmic droplet.

– The tail is 45 microns long, and is not bent or coiled.

Sperm Abnormalities

Sperm abnormalities are scored in four categories:

- For the head, abnormal characteristics include large, small, tapered, pyriform, amorphous, vacuolated, bicephalic, and acrosome defects.

- In the neck and midpiece, a distended or irregular midpiece, thin midpiece (no mitochondria), and bent or absent tail are abnormal.

- Abnormal tails may be short, multiple, hairpin, broken, or coiled.

- If there is a cytoplasmic droplet attached at the midpiece, the spermatozoon is considered immature.

Manual Assessment of Sperm Motility

Qualitative evaluation of forward motion:

0 = immotile.

1 = tail movement with no forward movement of the sperm.

2 = weak forward progression.

3 = active tail movement with good forward progression.

4 = vigorous tail movement with rapid forward progression.

TESTICULAR FACTORS OF INFERTILITY

Causes

Primary testicular problems may be chromosomal or nonchromosomal.

While chromosomal failure is usually caused by abnormalities of the sex chromosomes, autosomal disorders are also observed.

Chromosomal Abnormalities

Patients with azoospermia or severe oligospermia are more likely to have a chromosomal abnormality than infertile men with sperm density within the reference range.

– Klinefelter syndrome (47, XXY).

– XX male.

– XYY male.

– Noonan Syndrome.

– Mixed gonadal dysgenesis (45, X / 46, XY).

– Y-chromosome microdeletions.

– Bilateral anorchia (vanishing testis syndrome).

– Down syndrome.

– Myotonic muscular dystrophy.

– Congenital deficiency of testosterone production.

Nonchromosomal Testicular Failure

−Varicocele.

−Cryptorchidism.

−Androgen insensitivity syndrome (AIS).

−Sertoli-cell-only syndrome.

−Trauma.

−Orchitis.

−Chemotherapy.

−Radiotherapy.

−Idiopathic causes.

Investigations

The semen analysis is the cornerstone of the male infertility workup and includes assessment of the following:

−Semen quality.

−Semen volume (normal, 1.5-5 mL).

−Sperm density (normal, >15 million sperm/mL).

−Total sperm motility (normal, >40% of sperm having normal movement).

−Sperm morphology (lower limit for percentage of normal sperm is 4%).

- Signs of infection: increased number of white blood cells (WBCs) in the semen may be observed in patients with infectious or inflammatory processes.

- Other variables (eg, levels of zinc, citric acid, acid phosphatase, or alpha-glucosidase).

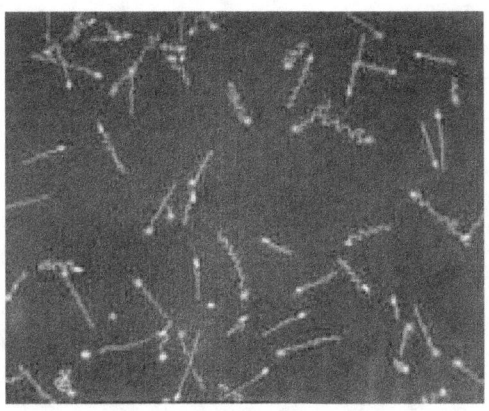

Semen Analysis

Other laboratory tests that may be helpful include the following:

- Antisperm antibody test.

- Genetic testing (karyotype, CFTR, AZF deletions if severe oligospermia (<5 million sperm/mL).

Imaging studies employed in this setting may include the following:

- Scrotal ultrasonography.

- Transrectal ultrasonography.

Indications for performing a postcoital test include semen hyperviscosity, increased or decreased semen volume with good sperm density, or unexplained infertility.

If the test result is normal, consider sperm function tests, such as the following:

−Capacitation assay.

−Acrosome reaction assay.

−Sperm penetration assay.

−Hypoosmotic swelling test.

−Inhibin B level.

−Vitality stains.

Treatment

Medical

The following causes of infertility, if identified, can often be treated by medical means:

−Poor semen quality or number.

−Infections.

−Antisperm antibodies.

−Lifestyle issues.

Surgical

– Varicocelectomy.

– Sperm retrieval techniques (MESA, PESA, TESE).

Assisted Reproduction Techniques (ART)

ART used to treat infertility include the following:

– Intrauterine insemination (IUI).

– In vitro fertilization (IVF).

– Gamete intrafallopian transfer (GIFT).

– Zygote intrafallopian transfer (ZIFT).

– Intracytoplasmic sperm injection (ICSI).

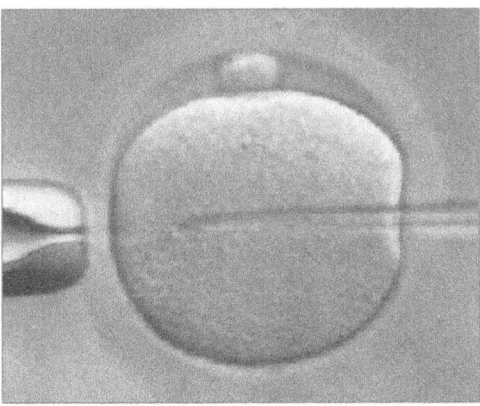

Intracytoplasmic Sperm Injection (ICSI)

Duct System

For each testis there is a duct system; the function of these ducts is testosterone-dependent.

The cells absorb fluid from the testis and remove particulate matter by endocytosis.

The epididymis is where sperm mature, concentrate and are stored for five to six days in this segment of the tract.

The vas deferens is a secondary storage site for spermatozoa; its epithelium has important absorptive and secretory functions.

The other components of the duct system are the ejaculatory duct and the urethra.

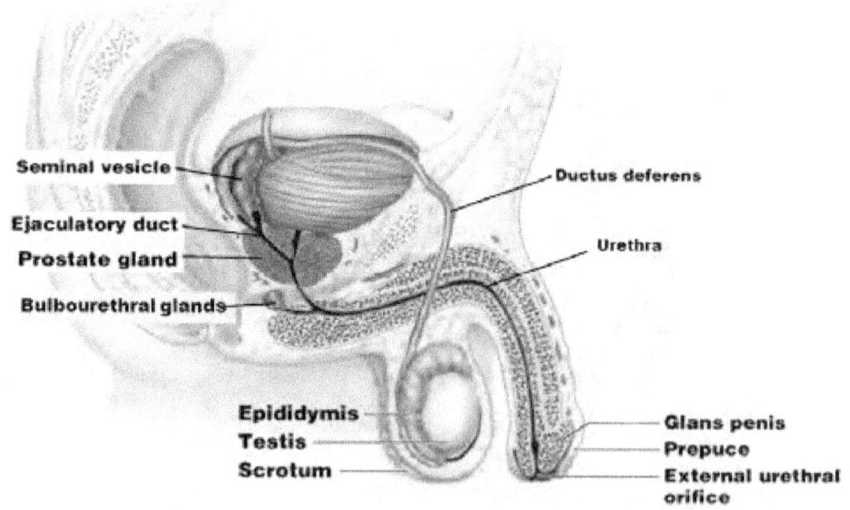

Duct System

Epididymis

The epididymis is a C-shaped structure lying intimately along the posterior border of each testis.

It includes an enlarged head, a body and a tail.

The tunica vaginalis covers the epididymis except at the posterior border.

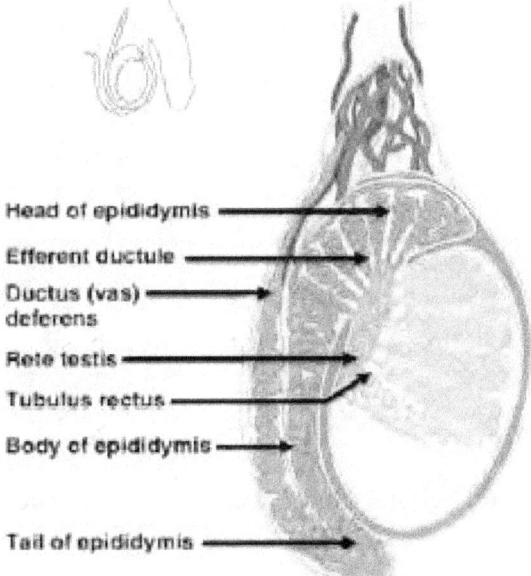

Epididymis

Vasculature and innervation of the epididymis is the same as for the testes.

Microscopic Anatomy

The main component of the epididymis is a tightly packed, tortuous duct approximately 6-m long and 400-µm in diameter.

The head consists of the most dense pack coils of efferent ductules, which are lined with ciliated columnar epithelium for transport of spermatozoa through the epididymis.

Functions

The epididymis is the major storage site of spermatozoa, which spend five to six days in this segment of the tract.

When sperm initially enter the epididymis, they are immotile and do not have the capacity to fertilize ova.

Tight junctions between epididymal epithelial cells maintain the blood-testis barrier, which is important for immune protection of sperm.

Epididymal fluid is enriched in potassium relative to semen and rich in glycerophosphorylcholine, a major energy source for spermatozoa .

The epididymis responds preferentially to dihydrotestosterone.

The epididymal histology and function change along its length:

– The initial segment connects with the rete testis and has tall columnar cells and a narrow lumen for major fluid absorption.

– In the caput, fluid becomes hyperosmotic and sperm attain motility.

– In the corpus, fertilizing potential is achieved with maturation of the sperm plasma membrane and sperm attain the ability to adhere to the zona pellucida of the ovum.

– In the cauda are cuboidal cells with a wide lumen for sperm storage; the luminal fluid becomes acidic as it moves from caput to cauda.

Ductus (Vas) Deferens

The ductus (vas) deferens is the continuation of the epididymis; it is 30-45-cm long and conveys sperm to the ejaculatory ducts.

The convoluted portion of ductus deferens becomes straighter (diameter, 2-3-mm) as it travels posterior to the testis and medial to the epididymis.

Subsequently, the ductus ascends on the posterior aspect of the spermatic cord until it reaches the deep inguinal ring, where it participates in the formation of spermatic cord and loops over the inferior epigastric artery.

At this point, the ductus travels along the lateral pelvic wall, medial to the distal ureter, along the posterior wall of the bladder until it reaches the seminal vesicles dorsal to the prostate.

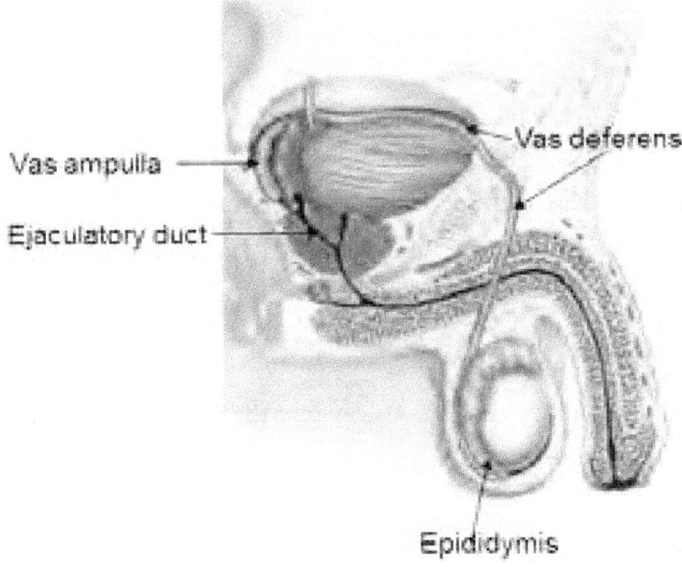

Ductus (Vas) Deferens

Each ductus deferens has an artery usually derived from the superior vesical artery (artery to the ductus).

Venous drainage is to the pelvic venous plexus.

Lymphatic drainage is to the external and internal iliac nodes.

Innervation is mainly sympathetic from the pelvic plexus.

Microscopic Anatomy

The ductus deferens is composed of pseudostratified columnar epithelium including columnar cells and basal cells.

The underlying lamina propria is dense with elastic fibers and the wall of the ductus contains three thick smooth muscle layers.

The outermost layer of adventitia is rich in blood vessels and nerves.

Functions

In the ductus deferens, there is rapid transport of sperm during ejaculation and slow transport and removal of excess sperm during sexual rest.

The proximal part of the vas is the site of vasectomy for contraception.

The distal part near the prostate, called the ampulla, stores sperm and empties into ejaculatory ducts that traverse the prostate gland to enter the urethra.

Spermatic Cord

The spermatic cord extends from the deep inguinal ring, through the inguinal canal to the testis.

The layers of the spermatic cord include (from outward to inward):

− External spermatic fascia (derived from the deep fascia of the external abdominal oblique muscle).

− Cremasteric fascia (derived from the internal oblique muscle).

− Internal spermatic fascia (derived from the transversalis fascia).

The structures that form the spermatic cord include:

− The ductus deferens and associated vasculature and nerves (posterior wall of the cord).

− The testicular artery.

− The pampiniform plexus, ultimately forming the testicular vein.

− The genital branch of the genitofemoral nerve.

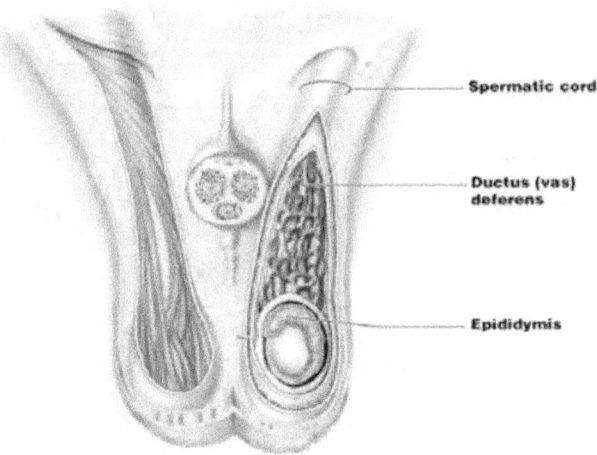

Spermatic cord

Ejaculatory Ducts

The ejaculatory ducts are 2-cm in length and derived from the union of the seminal vesicle and the ampulla of the vas deferens.

Each duct starts at the base of the prostate and terminates at the seminal colliculus (verumontanum).

The vasculature, innervation, and lymphatics of the ejaculatory ducts are the same as for the ductus deferens.

Urethra

The urethra stretches from the bladder to the tip of the glans penis, serving as a passage for urine and semen.

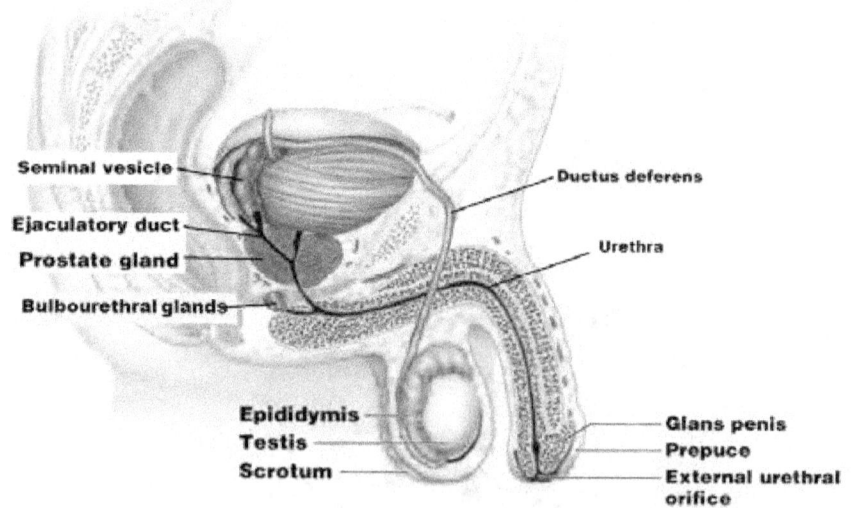

Male Urethra

The prostatic urethra extends vertically from the bladder neck, through the prostate before becoming the membranous urethra and before penetrating the perineal membrane; of note, the prostatic urethra contains the orifice of the ejaculatory ducts.

As the membranous urethra enters the deep perineal space, the urethra is surrounded by fibers of the external urethral sphincter, eventually entering the bulb of the corpus spongiosum, providing the orifice for the bulbourethral glands and subsequently becoming the penile urethra.

When the urethra reaches the glans penis the diameter diminishes to that of the external ostium, the least dilatable portion of the urethral canal.

Microscopic Anatomy

– The prostatic urethra is lined by transitional epithelium,

– The membranous urethra is lined by stratified columnar epithelium, and

– The penile urethra is initially stratified columnar epithelium and becomes stratified squamous epithelium at the fossa navicularis.

ACCESSORY GLANDS

Accessory glands include the seminal vesicle, prostate gland and bulbourethral glands.

The seminal vesicle provides precursor proteins responsible for semen coagulation, supplies fructose to nourish the ejaculated sperm and secretes prostaglandins that stimulate motility.

The prostate gland secretes proteolytic enzymes to liquefy coagulum after ejaculation, alkaline fluid to neutralize acidic vaginal secretions and the high zinc content is antimicrobial.

The bulbourethral glands, also known as Cowper's glands, secrete mucus for lubrication.

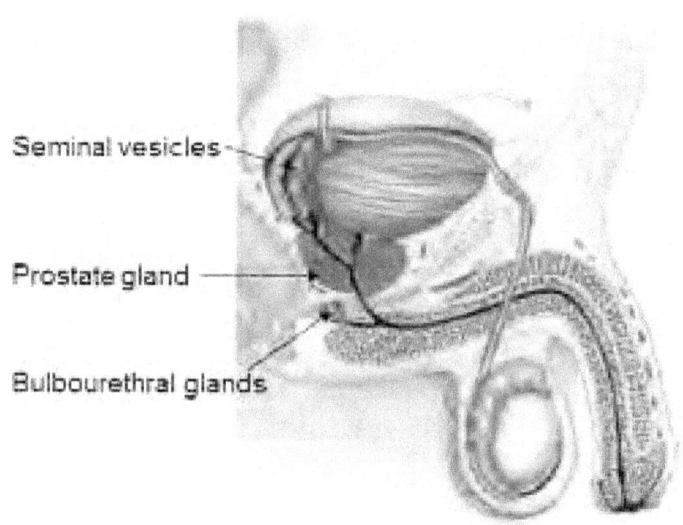

Accessory Glands

Seminal Vesicles

The 2 seminal vesicles are located between the bladder and the rectum and measure approximately 5 cm in length.

The anterior surface is in contact with the posterior wall of the bladder and the posterior surface is in contact with rectovesical fascia.

The ampulla of the ductus deferens lies medial to the seminal vesicles and the prostatic venous plexus lies laterally.

Arterial blood supply to the seminal vesicles includes branches from the inferior vesical and middle rectal arteries, while venous and lymphatic drainage accompanies these arteries.

The inferior division of the hypogastric plexus provides innervation to the seminal vesicles.

Microscopic Anatomy

The seminal vesicles are tubulosaccular glands consisting of connective tissue and secretory epithelium projecting into the lumen of the gland.

The epithelium is pseudostratified with basal and columnar cells, while the wall of the vesicle is consistent with a thick wall of smooth muscle.

Functions

The seminal vesicles, which are testosterone-dependent, have important secretory function, but they have little storage capacity.

They produce a very alkaline secretion and fibrin, which is responsible for coagulation of semen after ejaculation.

Prostate

The prostate gland is an ovoid structure encompassing the proximal portion of the urethra and

It is approximately 2.5-3.0 cm by 4.0-4.5 cm, and normally weighing 20-25 g.

Relations of the prostate gland:

– The base of the prostate is in contact with the bladder.

– The apex is superior to the perineal membrane.

– The anterior border is in contact with the vesicoprostatic plexus.

– The posterior border is separated from the anterior surface of the rectum by the rectovesical (Denonvilliers) fascia.

– The lateral border is in contact with the levator ani and the prostatic venous plexus.

– Fibers of the external urethral sphincter surround the prostate.

The arterial supply to the prostate gland is derived from the inferior vesical artery and branches of the middle rectal artery.

Venous drainage of the prostate forms the prostatic plexus, which eventually drains into the internal iliac vein.

Lymphatic drainage flows to the internal iliac nodes.

Innervation is derived from the inferior portion of the hypogastric plexus, primarily to the connective tissue surrounding the gland.

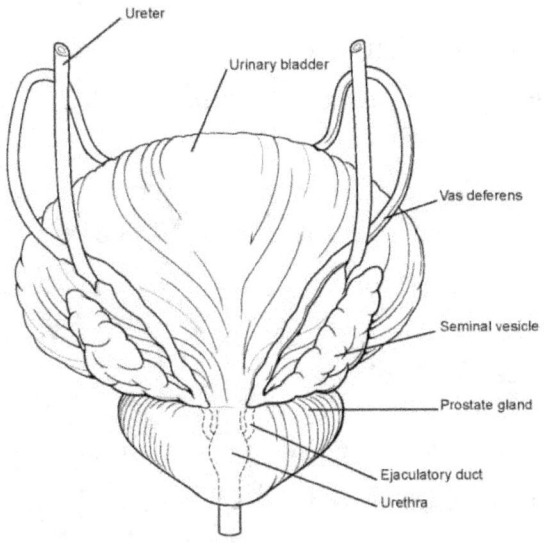

Prostate Gland

Microscopic Anatomy

The prostate is traditionally divided into three concentric zones:

– The peripheral zone constitutes 70% of the prostate and contains the tubuloalveolar glands of the organ.

– The central zone constitutes 25% and contains submucosal glands.

– The transitional zone constitutes 5% of the prostate.

The tubuloalveolar glands are embedded in a fibrous stroma and open through branching ducts in the prostatic urethra.

The secretory nature of the epithelium is evident as it consists of pseudostratified epithelium containing basal and secretory cells.

Functions

The prostate gland, which is dihydrotestosterone-dependent, produces a slightly acidic (pH 6.5), colorless, thin secretion, rich in minerals and sodium.

The prostate gland produces the enzyme fibrinolysin, which degrades the fibrin clot in coagulated semen.

Bulbourethral Glands

The bilateral bulbourethral glands are 2 cm in diameter and lie lateral to the membranous urethra and are enclosed by the external urethral sphincter.

The excretory duct of the gland penetrates the perineal membrane and opens within the bulbar urethra.

Vasculature, lymphatic drainage, and innervation are generally the same as for the seminal vesicles.

The bulbourethral glands secrete mucus for lubrication during sexual intercourse.

PENIS

The penis is made up of an attached root and a pendulous body.

The root consists of two crura and the bulb - 3 bodies of erectile tissue attached to the pubic arch (crura) and perineal membrane (bulb).

Near the border of the pubic sypmphysis the bilateral crura continue as the corpora cavernosa throughout the body of the penis.

The bulb lies between the two crura, narrows anteriorly and continues as the corpus spongiosum.

The corpora cavernosa are enveloped in a thick fibrous tunica albuginea, which is comprised of a longitudinal running superficial fibers and a deep layer of circular oriented fibers.

The corpus spongiosum is penetrated by the urethra as it traverses the body of the penis.

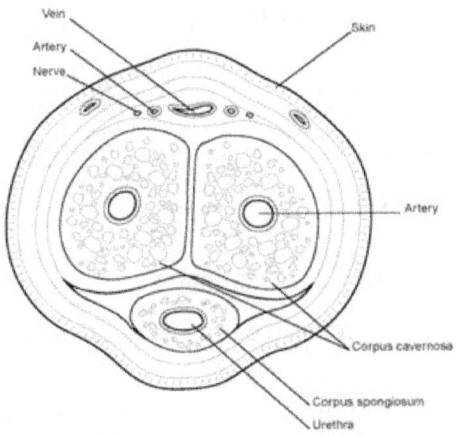

Cross-sectional Anatomy of the Penis

The superficial penile fascia includes loose connective tissue intertwined with dartos muscle fibers.

The deep penile fascia, or Buck's fascia, is a tough fascial layer that encompasses both corpora cavernosa and the corporus spongiosum.

The skin of the penis is thin; the corona of the penis is where the skin folds to become the prepuce (foreskin), enveloping the glans penis.

The vasculature of the penis is extensive.

The perineal artery (a branch of the internal pudendal artery) together with the posterior scrotal artery and the inferior rectal artery supply tissues from the bulb of the penis to the anus.

The artery of the bulb of the penis, from the internal pudendal, penetrates the penile bulb and subsequently supplies the corpus spongiosum.

The deep artery of the penis, one of two terminal branches of the internal pudendal artery, enters the crus of the penis and continues through the length of the bilateral corpus cavernosum.

The other terminal branch of the internal pudendal artery is the dorsal artery of the penis running along the dorsal surface of the penis supplying the penile skin and the glans penis.

The venous drainage of the penis includes the veins draining the corpora cavernosa, which subsequently drains into the circumflex veins.

These veins receive venous blood from the corpus spongiosum on the ventral aspect of the penis and wrap around the penis to drain into the deep dorsal vein.

The superficial dorsal vein drains the penile skin and prepuce before draining via the superficial external pudendal vein into the external pudendal veins.

The deep dorsal vein further drains blood from the glans penis and corpora cavernosa before joining the prostatic venous plexus.

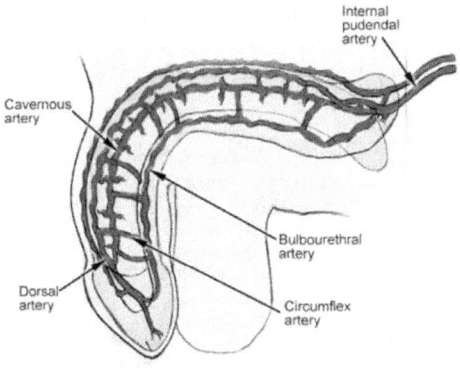

Arterial Supply of the Penis

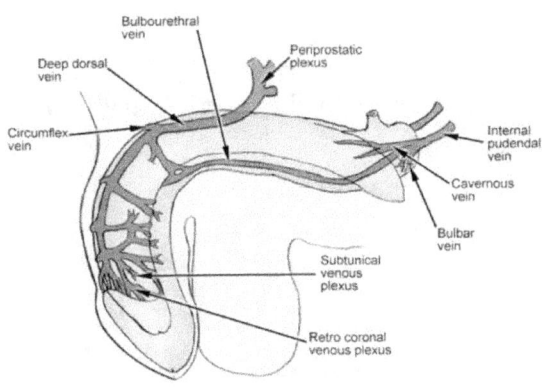

Venous Drainage of the Penis

The lymphatic drainage of the penis encompasses three locations:

– The superficial inguinal nodes (penile skin).

– Deep inguinal and external iliac nodes (glans penis).

– Internal iliac nodes (erectile tissue and urethra).

Sensory innervation to the penile skin is through the dorsal nerve of the penis, one of the terminal branches of the pudendal nerve.

Autonomic innervation includes both sympathetic and parasympathetic aspects to the corpora cavernosum via the cavernous nerves.

The sympathetic fibers originate at the level of T11-T12 and the parasympathetic fibers originate from the pelvic plexus at S2-S4.

Microscopic Anatomy

The erectile bodies of the penis are composed of fibroelastic connective tissue, smooth muscle and a network of vascular sinuses lined with endothelium.

The sinuses are continuous with the arteries that supply them and the veins that drain them.

ERECTION AND EJACULATION

In the relaxed state, the central arteries in the cavernosa are constricted, limiting blood inflow; blood flows through sinusoids, and out through veins.

In the aroused state, impulses from the brain and local nerves cause the central arteries to dilate and the muscles of the corpora cavernosa to relax.

The blood fills the sinusoids to compress the veins, reducing venous outflow and causing an erection.

As the tunica albuginea expands it compresses exiting veins to help trap blood in the corpora cavernosa, thereby sustaining the erection.

Emission is a sympathetic and parasympathetic (S2-S4) event causing peristaltic waves up the vas deferens and contractions from the seminal vesicles and prostate gland to expel contents to the prostatic urethra.

Ejaculation is expulsion of the semen in the prostatic urethra distally down the urethra.

Ejaculation occurs by expulsion of the contents of the bulbourethral glands, followed by the fluid from the epididymis and prostate, accounting for about 30% of volume and the highest sperm concentration.

Lastly, the seminal vesicles empty and produce the largest portion of the seminal volume.

Semen is an admixture of sperm cells and secretions from the male accessory sex glands that combine at the time of ejaculation.

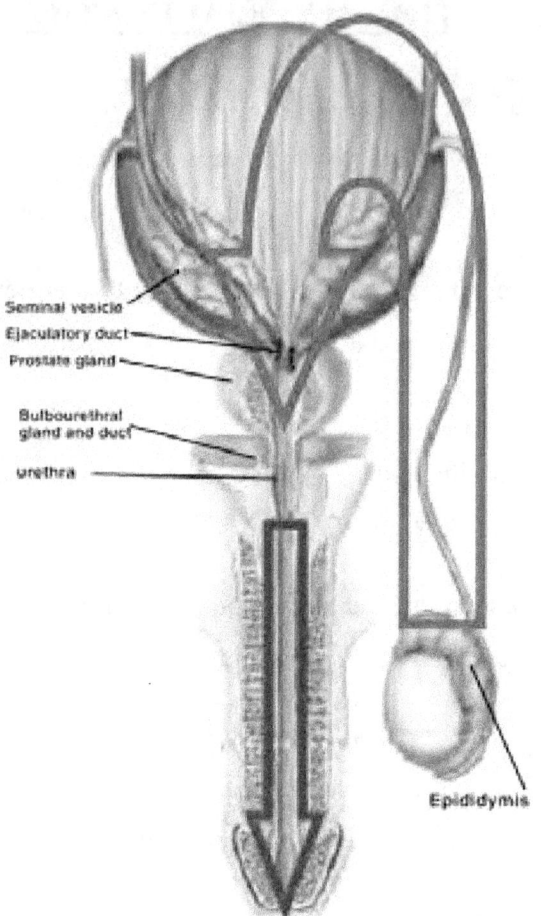

Mechanism of Ejaculation

POSTTESTICULAR FACTORS OF INFERTILITY

Causes

Posttesticular causes of infertility include problems with sperm transportation through the ductal system, either congenital or acquired.

Additionally, the sperm may be unable to cross the cervical mucus or may have ultrastructural abnormalities.

− Congenital blockage of the ductal system.

− Congenital bilateral absence of the vas deferens (CBAVD).

− Acquired ductal obstruction.

− Antisperm antibodies.

− Ejaculatory duct obstruction.

− Ejaculatory disorders.

− Erectile dysfunction.

Investigations

− Testicular biopsy is indicated in azoospermic men with a normal-sized testis and normal findings on hormonal studies to evaluate for ductal obstruction and to retrieve sperm.

− Vasography.

− Antisperm antibodies.

Treatment

Medical

– Infections.

– Retrograde ejaculation.

Surgical

– Vasovasostomy or vasoepididymostomy.

– Transurethral resection of the ejaculatory ducts.

– Sperm retrieval techniques (MESA, PESA, TESE).

Assisted Reproduction Techniques (ART)

– Intracytoplasmic sperm injection (ICSI).

REFERENCES

- Brugh V, Lipshultz L. Male factor infertility. Medical Clinics of North America. 2004; 88: 367-85.

- Chung K. Gross Anatomy. 4th ed. Philadelphia: Lippincott Williams & Wilkins; 2000.

- Drake R, Vogl A, Mitchell A. Gray's Anatomy for Student's. 2nd ed. Philadelphia: Churchill Livingstone Elsevier; 2010.

- Gillen-water J, Grayhack J, Howards S, et al, editors. Adult and pediatric urology. 4th ed. London: Lippincott. Williams & Wilkins; 2002.

- Gray H. Anatomy, Descriptive and Surgical. The Unabridged Gray's Anatomy. Philadelphia: Running Press; 1999.

- Hirsh A. Male subfertility. BMJ. 2003; 327: 669-72.

- Junqueira L, Carneiro J, Kelley R. Basic Histology. 9th ed. Stamford, Connecticut: Appleton & Lange; 1998.

- Katz V, Lentz G, Lobo R, et al. Comprehensive Gynecology. 5th ed. Philadelphia: Mosby Elsevier; 2007.

- Loukas M, Colburn G, Abrahams P, et al. Gray's Anatomy Review. Philadelphia: Churchill Livingstone Elsevier; 2010.

- Neill J. Knobil and Neill's Physiology of Reproduction. 3rd ed. St. Louis, MO: Elsevier; 2006.

- Ovalle W, Nahirney P. Netter's Eseential Histology. Philadelphia: Sauders Elsevier; 2007.

- Practice Committee of the American Society for Reproductive Medicine. Optimal evaluation of the infertile male. Fertil Steril. 2006; 86: S202-9.

References

- Practice Committee of the American Society for Reproductive Medicine. Optimal evaluation of the infertile female. Fertil Steril. 2006; 86: S264-7.

- Rotterdam ESHRE/ASRM-Sponsored PCOS Consensus Workshop Group. Revised 2003 consensus on diagnostic criteria and long-term health risks related to polycystic ovary syndrome. Fertil Steril. 2004; 81: 19-25.

- Sadler T. Langman's Medical Embryology. 11th ed. Baltimore, Maryland: Lippincott Williams & Wilkins; 2010.

- Speroff L, Fritz M, eds. Clinical Gynecologic Endocrinology and Infertility, 7th ed. Philadelphia: Lippincot, Williams & Wilkins, 2005.

- Standring S. Gray's Anatomy. 40th ed. Edinburgh: Churchill Livingstone Elsevier; 2008.

- Wein A. Campbell-Walsh Urology. 9th ed. Philadelphia: Saunders Elsevier; 2007.

- World Health Organization. WHO Laboratory Manual for the Examination and Processing of Human Semen. 5th Edition. Geneva, Switzerland: WHO; 2010.

www.ingramcontent.com/pod-product-compliance
Lightning Source LLC
Chambersburg PA
CBHW072014230526
45468CB00021B/1507